EXPERIMENTAL RESEARCHES

ON THE

CAUSES AND NATURE

OF

CATARRHUS ÆSTIVUS.

EXPERIMENTAL RESEARCHES

ON THE

CAUSES AND NATURE

OF

CATARRHUS ÆSTIVUS

(HAY-FEVER OR HAY-ASTHMA).

BY

CHARLES H. BLACKLEY, M.R.C.S. Eng.

OXFORD HISTORICAL BOOKS
Abingdon 1988

OXFORD HISTORICAL BOOKS
Harrowdown, Longworth,
Abingdon, Oxon OX13 5ET,
England

First published 1873 by Baillière Tindall and Cox. This facsimile of the first edition is produced with the kind permission of their successors, Baillière Tindall of London.

ISBN 1 871395 00 3

Printed in Great Britain

PREFACE.

HAY-FEVER has, in England, been for some years attracting a considerable share of attention amongst the members of the medical profession and also in a less degree amongst those who are unconnected with the profession. Hitherto, however, its causes and, to some extent, its real nature have been but imperfectly understood.

In the investigations which are detailed in the following pages the object has been to test, by actual experiment, the validity of the opinions held on the causes of the disease, as well as to collect additional information upon points which were uncertain or doubtful, and thus to help to clear up some of the obscurities which have rested upon the subject. Being for the most part a record of the personal experience gained in following out the inquiry, the observations are not intended to settle the question of cause for all cases of the disorder. Nevertheless I believe that the results of the experiments, along with the evidence collected from other sources, fully warrant the conclusion that the cases which are due to any other cause than that named are so few in number that they may be considered mere exceptions to a general rule.

To those members of the profession who have studied hay-fever and have formed definite opinions upon it, it will appear that the mode in which the subject is treated is unnecessarily minute, but to those who are imperfectly acquainted with the disease, or to whom it is entirely new, it will not appear that too much detail has been given. Even in this country, where the disorder probably had its commencement and where it is still more common than in any other part of Europe, there are medical men to be found who know very little about it; and on the Continent there are still some to be found who have never even heard of the disease. To such as these especially the details I have given will not be uninteresting.

It is a matter of regret to me, and I have no doubt will be to some of my readers, that I have not been able to speak at length and with some degree of certainty and precision upon the treatment of hay-fever. A determination to adhere as closely as possible to the statement of such facts as my own experience would enable me to vouch for, compels me to say that treatment by medicines has so far, in my hands, been very unsatisfactory; nor do I think that it would have been found to be any more successful in the hands of those who *seem* to have been more fortunate, if a strictly logical method of testing the efficacy of treatment had been followed.

I do not, however, despair of a specific being found for hay-fever, and offer the following pages as a contribution which it is hoped may assist somewhat in the search for the appropriate remedy.

In the course of the enquiry I have been indebted to several medical friends for their kindness in calling my attention to anything which bore upon the subject I had in hand, and also for procuring for me books and papers relating to hay-fever, as well as for other important services rendered during the time the investigations have been in progress.

From some non-professional friends also I have received very valuable aid. To my friend Mr. Herman G. Kindt,* I am especially indebted for his kindness in translating for me the greater portion of the work of Professor Phœbus as well as for other valuable assistance which he gave in the early part of the experiments. To my friend Mr. James Lord† I am also under great obligation for the help he gave me in nearly all the experiments at high altitudes. To each and all of these friends I tender my most sincere thanks.

CHAS. H. BLACKLEY.

STRETFORD ROAD, MANCHESTER;
    April 5th, 1873.

---

* Now of Neustrelitz, Germany.
† Of Whalley Range, Manchester.

DIRECTIONS TO THE BINDER.

Table I is to face page 129.
Table II   „   139.

Plate I   „   97.
Plates II and III } are to be placed between pages 118 and 119.
Plate IV is to face page 122.
Plate V   „   140.
Plate VI   „   145.
Plate VII   „   149.

ERRATA.

At § 27, line 11, for "or indeed," read "*nor indeed.*"
„ § 166, „ 1, for "If his theory was," read "*If his theory were.*"
„ § 195, „ 7, for "§ 189," read "§ 192."
„ § 224, „ 9, for "was copious," read "*was a copious.*"

TABLE OF CONTENTS.

CHAPTER I.
INTRODUCTION . . . . PAGE 1

CHAPTER II.
A REVIEW OF THE OPINIONS HELD ON THE CAUSES OF HAY-FEVER . 12

CHAPTER III.
EXPERIMENTS WITH, AND OBSERVATIONS ON, THE PRESUMED CAUSES OF HAY-FEVER 49

CHAPTER IV.
ON THE QUANTITY OF POLLEN FOUND FLOATING IN THE ATMOSPHERE DURING THE PREVALENCE OF HAY-FEVER, AND ON ITS RELATION TO THE INTENSITY OF THE SYMPTOMS 115

CHAPTER V.
ON THE GREATER PREVALENCE OF HAY-FEVER, AND ON THE INCREASE OF ITS PREDISPOSING AND EXCITING CAUSES . . . 154

CHAPTER VI.
ON THE SYMPTOMS AND NATURE OF HAY-FEVER . . . 163

EXPERIMENTAL RESEARCHES

ON THE

NATURE AND CAUSES OF CATARRHUS ÆSTIVUS

(HAY-FEVER, OR HAY-ASTHMA).

CHAPTER I.

INTRODUCTION.

§ 1. At no period in the history of medicine has the investigation of the causes of disease been carried on more assiduously than it is at the present day. Such is the magnitude of the work, however, and so great are the difficulties which are inseparable from it, that comparatively little has yet been accomplished, and it is still, practically, one of the widest and also one of the least exhausted fields of inquiry in the whole domain of science.

It is not that it can furnish occupation to the thoughtful and curious mind merely, or that it offers an almost unbounded *terra incognita* to the scientific explorer who desires to traverse unknown regions, that it ought to invite our attention and make us desirous of laying bare its secrets. It has wider and more direct and intimate relations to the physical well-being of mankind than any question of mere abstract science can give, and it will be readily admitted that the successful elucidation of the etiology of disease is fraught with consequences the value of which it is scarcely possible to estimate. It is, moreover, probable that in this field of research there are to be found some of the brightest laurels which can be won by the scientific discoverer.

§ 2. Whether we accept the germ theory of disease, and regard these germs as portions of organic matter, which have a separate and independent existence and as capable of growth and multiplication, within the organism, to an extent at present undetermined, or accept what has lately been designated the "physical theory," and maintain that the causes of communicable diseases do not possess any of the characteristics of germs, we shall still have to admit that disease is, in a large number of instances, the result of the operation of two principal factors:—The one being a condition of the animal body which permits the development of disease in that organism—the other that of some agent external to the body, which becomes operative whenever there is present the condition above named, or whenever this external agent is in sufficient quantity to overcome the resistance which every organ is, in a state of health, able to offer to that which is inimical to the due performance of its functions.

§ 3. The first condition named, though often varying, is probably always present, in a greater or lesser degree, even in the most healthy subject. The second, in like manner, is probably as variable as the first, and, though possibly always present in the larger centres of modern civilisation, is ever changing in its quantity or its power.

§ 4. The essential nature of that state of the organism which gives a proclivity to disease, and permits external agents to act upon the animal body, so as to produce morbid conditions, may never be fully known to us; and it may be that, with our present means of research, the active causes of many of our most formidable maladies will elude our grasp for long years to come. There are, however, some of the more simple and less fatal diseases in which, by an improved method of study, we may hope to obtain a better knowledge than we now possess of the nature and *modus operandi* of those external agents which act as exciting causes; and it is, perhaps, in searching for such that we shall most easily learn very important lessons in studying the etiology of disease.

§ 5. The importance of this study has been noticed by some authors who have long since passed away. One of these, who wrote in the early part of the present century, in speaking of the study and practice of the art of medicine, very forcibly says :—

"As it is physical influences with which we have chiefly to do in medicine, the main and ultimate object in cultivating this art must consist in ascertaining the agency of external objects, whether salutary or noxious, on the living body, and in applying these, or avoiding them, so as to obtain the desired result, either of preventing the occurrence of disease or of converting the state of disease into that of health. It is to the extent and correctness of our knowledge of these agencies that the perfection of the art of physic must consist."*

The remarks made by the illustrious author just quoted apply with considerable force to the study of the malady which is the subject of the inquiries and experiments described in the following pages.

§ 6. This disorder is an example of those which are mild and non-fatal in their character, and on this account offers opportunities for investigating it with comparative safety.

Many able authors have written upon hay-fever, and considerable effort has been made to explain and to account for its phenomena, but, so far, there has been but little progress made towards a complete understanding of these ; nor have we yet made much, if any, advance towards obtaining a remedy on which we can depend as an effectual means of cure.

§ 7. Hay-fever or hay-asthma was first known in this country, and may indeed be said to have had its birth-place in England. It was first described by Bostock in the year 1819. In a paper read before the Medico-Chirurgical Society of London he gave an account of a case which was termed "A case of the Periodical Affection of the Eyes and Chest,"† and which was in reality a description of his own

---

* *Medical Logick*, by Sir Gilbert Blane. London, 1819.

† "Case of a Periodical Affection of the Eyes and Chest," by John Bostock, M.D. *Medico-Chirurgical Transactions*, London, 1819, vol. x, part i, pp. 161—165.

case. Heberden had previously mentioned* such a catarrh as is understood to have been what is now termed hay-fever, but he does not seem to have known anything of its real nature. Cullen also remarks that in some persons asthmatic fits are more frequent in summer, and more particularly during the dog-days, than at other colder seasons of the year. In 1828 Dr. Bostock read a second paper† on this subject before the above-named society, and gave a more lengthy and exact account of the symptoms of the disease.

§ 8. In the time which had elapsed between the reading of his first and second papers Bostock had either seen or had received " distinct accounts of eighteen cases," besides about ten others in which " the accounts were less perfect." In the latter communication the disorder was designated " Catarrhus æstivus " or " Summer catarrh." It is by this name it has since been more or less known among medical men, but from the circumstance of its having been noticed that it commonly came on during the hay-season it has obtained, among the laity, the name of hay-fever or hay-asthma, and I am inclined to believe that these names will be found to be the most appropriate of any yet used.

§ 9. The literature of the disease was, up to a comparatively recent period, very scanty. Bostock's first paper was published, as stated above, in 1819, and between this and his second communication in 1828 there was an interval of nine years, in which no other notice of the disease appeared in a printed form.

§ 10. In 1828 Dr. Macculloch‡ mentioned the disease, and in speaking of its causes says, " It is produced by hot-houses or green-houses, and in the public estimation it is particularly caused by hay-fields."

§ 11. In 1829 Mr. W. Gordon published his " Observa-

---

* *Commentary on the History and Cure of Diseases.* 4th edition. London, 1816. Chap. " Destillatio," p. 113.

† " On Catarrhus Æstivus, or Summer Catarrh," by Thos. Bostock, M.D. *Medico-Chirurgical Transactions*, 1828, vol. xii, p. 437—446.

‡ *An Essay on the Remittent and Intermittent Diseases*, by Dr. John Macculloch, London, 1828, vol. i, pp. 394—397.

tions on the Nature, Cause, and Treatment of Hay-Asthma."*

§ 12. In 1830 Mr. Augustus Præter published a short notice of a case he had seen in Paris some years before.

§ 13. In 1831 Dr. Elliotson noticed the disease in his lectures, and again in 1833 he gave a more lengthened account of the malady.

§ 14. From this latter period there was again an interval of ten years during which there was not anything of a special character published on hay-fever.

§ 15. Since the time just mentioned the subject has gradually excited increased interest amongst the laity and also amongst the members of the medical profession; and it would seem that there are now a greater number of cases to be met with than there were formerly. Perhaps this may, in part, be due to the increased attention, directed to the disease, having had the effect of bringing the cases, which do occur, much more distinctly under the notice of medical men than they have been brought at any previous period; but it may also be, in part, accounted for by the greater prevalence of those conditions which act as predisposing and exciting causes.

§ 16. This increased interest in the disease has shown itself in the publication of numerous articles on it in the periodical medical literature, and in the works of various writers on systematic medicine, both on the continent and in this country. There have also been several treatises published in a separate form during the last few years. Among the principal of those which have been published in this country may be mentioned those of Dr. Abbotts Smith,† Dr. Pirrie,‡ and Dr. G. Moore.§ Although the disease is more prevalent in England than in any other part of the

---

* "Observations on the Nature, Cause, and Treatment of Hay Asthma," by Wm. Gordon, M.R.C.S. Edin. *London Med. Gazette*, 1829, vol. iv, pp. 266—269.

† *Observations on Hay Fever, Hay Asthma, or Summer Catarrh,* by Wm Abbotts Smith, M.D., M.R.C.P.Lond. London, 1865. 2nd edition.

‡ *On Hay Asthma, or the Affection termed Hay Fever,* by Wm. Pirrie, M.D., &c. &c. London, 1867.

§ *Hay Fever, or Summer Catarrh : its Causes, Symptoms, Prevention, and Treatment,* by George Moore, M.D. London, 1869.

world, it is to a German author (Dr. Phœbus, professor of medicine at Giessen) that we are indebted for the best monograph * that has yet appeared on hay-fever.†

§ 17. In speaking of the disease having been brought so recently under notice Bostock says:—

"One of the most remarkable circumstances respecting the complaint is its not having been noticed as a special affection until the last ten or twelve years. Except a single observation of Heberden's I have not met with anything that can be said to refer to it in any author, either ancient or modern."‡

As far as the researches into the literature of the disease up to the present time have shown, there does not appear to have been any notice of it previous to that which is here mentioned by Bostock.

§ 18. Considering the high character which the physicians of that day bore as acute observers, it seems strange, at first sight, if the disease did exist, that it should not have been recognised and described by them. Whether the malady had been only recently developed when Heberden first mentioned it, or whether it was then of much older standing, we may not now be able to ascertain.

19. Dr. Copland tells us that, up to the time of Sydenham, rheumatism and gout had been regarded as one and the same disorder. These forms of disease have less similarity and are more distinct in their characters than are the catarrhal form of hay-fever and common coryza; whilst in the asthmatic form of hay-fever it is impossible to distinguish between the latter and common asthma except by determining what the exciting cause is.§ It may not, therefore, seem so remarkable that hay-fever may have been long mistaken for the ordinary form of coryza or of asthma; and when we consider that there are not wanting instances of even medical men having been affected

---

* *Der Typische Frühsommer Katarrh oder das sogenannte Heufieber, Heu-asthma,* von Philipp Phœbus, M.D., &c. &c. Giessen, 1862.

† It is to this work that I am indebted for the names of all the foreign authors, and for those of several English authors, who have written on hay-fever.

‡ This remark occurs in Bostock's second paper, published in 1828.

§ This remark applies only to the purely asthmatic form of the disorder.

by this malady, and who have not become fully aware of its nature until they had suffered from it for some time, it may be considered highly probable that it had occurred in isolated cases long prior to the time when it was first noticed by medical authors.

§ 20. Hay-fever is said to be an aristocratic disease, and there can be no doubt that, if it is not almost wholly confined to the upper classes of society, it is rarely, if ever, met with but among the educated. Dr. Phœbus and other writers speak of cases which have occurred among the working part of the population. I have myself never seen or had any such cases brought under my notice; and I think it is tolerably certain that, if they occur at all, they do so but very seldom. I have met with cases of chronic catarrh among the working classes which seemed at first sight to resemble hay-fever, but when tested in the manner described in my experiments, the patients were found not to be amenable to the same influences as are those individuals who suffer from the genuine disease.

§ 21. In perusing the literature of hay-fever one is struck with the great variety of opinion which prevails upon its causes, and also, in some degree, upon its nature, but more especially with the small amount of success which has apparently attended its treatment. This want of unanimity of opinion on its causes, and the want of success in its treatment, have perhaps been the most marked where medical men themselves have been the subjects of the malady; whilst, on the other hand, singular as it may appear, those who seem to have been the most fortunate in treating others have themselves never suffered from the disorder.

This diversity of opinion and the failure which has attended the efforts to cure the disorder may be, and probably are, to some extent, due to the absence of any attempt at proving by inductive methods of experimentation the precise nature of its causes, and also to not endeavouring to ascertain by the same means the relative value of the remedies used in its treatment; and, to use the words of a recent writer, it is "a matter of astonishment that greater efforts have not been made to elucidate the doubtful points relating to its history, causes, and treatment, and thus to obtain a more certain guide to the relief or cure of the disease."*

§ 22. In the course of my reading on this subject I became convinced that something more needed to be done, than had already been accomplished, before we could say that we had got hold of the "sum of the facts" to which the disease owes its existence. It seemed as if we had hitherto failed to grasp the idea that "the cause cannot be anything which is present in other cases where the given effect is not produced, unless the presence of some counteracting cause shall appear to account for its non-production."†

§ 23. In regard also to the mass of evidence already collected there seemed to be a great need of this being sifted and re-arranged on a more logical method; and, more than all, there appeared to be a necessity for a collection of additional facts in order that we might fill up the missing links in the chain of evidence, so as to give us the means of a closer and more correct generalisation.

The annual recurrence of the malady at a given period of the year, the almost certain departure of it after a given time, the entire freedom from it which most patients enjoy for the greater part of the year, the absence of any dangerous symptoms, except in rare cases, as well as the non-occurrence of sequelæ of a serious character, seem to offer opportunities for safe experimentation such as are rarely found in any other complaint, whilst the presumed exciting causes are such as to present no great obstacle to their being fairly tested during the intervals of freedom from the disorder.

§ 24. If any reason needed to be given for these investigations having been undertaken by me, it is partly furnished in the remarks made above, but principally by the circumstance that I have myself been a sufferer from this curious malady for more than twenty years.

Although I had in the earlier years of my attacks of hay-fever carefully read all the then very scanty literature of the disease, I had not been able to form any very definite and

---

* Preface to Dr. Abbotts Smith's first edition of his work on *Hay-Fever*.
† Archbishop Thomson's *Outline of the Laws of Thought*.

settled notion of the nature of the cause. I was inclined to regard heat as the principal exciting cause, but my experience did not quite coincide with the opinions of those who had written on the disorder, and this experience had, unfortunately, compelled me to come to the conclusion that, until something more was known than I had learned from the writings of others or from my own previous observations, there was no chance of escape from the annual torment. I had thus a personal interest in getting a more thorough knowledge than I then possessed of all the phenomena of hay-fever; and whilst I was in this way furnished with a good and sufficient reason for commencing the investigations, the annoyance caused by the annual attacks acted as a powerful stimulus to exertion in making these as complete as my somewhat limited time and opportunities would permit.

§ 25. The experiments, which I have to describe in a succeeding chapter, were commenced in the year 1859, but owing to various circumstances, which were not controllable at the time, proceeded very slowly for some years. This delay was in some measure owing to the difficulty there was in sparing sufficient time for a lengthened and uninterrupted course of observations during some of the spring and summer months. For the purposes I had in view, it was absolutely necessary that a number of observations should be made each day during the period named, and that these should commence some time before the grass came into flower, and be continued until it had been all gathered in. It was also necessary that some person who suffered from hay-fever should be exposed during a portion of the day, at least, to the influences which might prevail in the district in which the observations were taken, and that the symptoms generated by such exposure should be registered daily. It would have been more satisfactory, and would have brought out more exact results, if the patient to be experimented upon could have been kept within a short radius of the spot selected for the first series of experiments; but as this would have involved a sort of imprisonment for at least ten weeks, it was impossible for me to follow out the investigation in this very precise manner. What, however, the observations have lacked in this respect, I have endeavoured to some extent to make up for by following out the inquiry under varying circumstances and in different districts. It would also have been well if I could have had the co-operation of some other individual who, like myself, was a sufferer from hay-fever. In two attempts which I made to induce others to undertake experiments upon themselves I failed, although these were of a very limited and simple character.

§ 26. There is one part of the subject which would well repay careful investigation, viz., the chemical constitution of the pollen of various plants, and especially those of the order Graminaceæ. Into this I have not been able to enter, but I cannot doubt that it would be well worth the time and trouble which would have to be expended on such an inquiry, if some able chemist would take up the matter and ascertain all that can be known of the constituents of pollen.

§ 27. In the first years of the disease, in my own case, it had more than once happened that, when some particular plan of treatment was being pursued, this would seem for a time to be successful in mitigating the severity of the symptoms, and, in some instances, in apparently curing the malady; but suddenly, and without any change in the treatment, there would be a complete relapse, and the condition would become as bad as before. Subsequent experience, in seasons when the disease was present, and when no treatment of any kind was being used, convinced me that these variations were not due to, or indeed, in any degree, influenced by the treatment adopted, but that they were probably the result of a variation in the *quantity* or *quality* of the causes of the malady, whatever these might be.

§ 28. It seemed, therefore, to be highly important that not only the *nature* of the cause of this disease should be discovered, but that we should have the means of measuring its variations in *quantity* as well as *quality*; and that we should particularly study those circumstances which lead to these variations. There was also another question to which it was important to obtain an answer if possible, viz., whether in any individual case the disease owned only one exciting cause, or whether it had a plurality of causes.

Until the latter questions were satisfactorily settled it was clear that any effort to gain relief, by avoiding the one supposed cause, might be completely frustrated by the patient unwittingly putting himself under the influence of other hostile circumstances. But once accomplish these objects, and we should not only be better able to gain relief by avoiding the cause, but we should have the means of erecting a standard by which we should be able to estimate the value of the remedies used in the cure of the disorder. So long, however, as we were ignorant of the real nature of the influences which give rise to the morbid conditions and of the possible rates of their variation, we were constantly liable to be misled in our estimate of the efficacy of the remedies used.

§ 29. It was with the hope of accomplishing something in the direction indicated that these experiments were commenced. The main object was to find out what were the exciting causes of the attacks in my own case; but as an examination of the records of other cases showed me that in its symptoms, and in the conditions which seemed to give rise to these, my own case was almost identical with a very large majority of those I had investigated, it appeared to be highly probable that if I succeeded in ascertaining the cause in my own case, I should also be doing the same thing for a large number of other patients. If, after making the attempt, I found that I was not able to do satisfactorily all that I have indicated above, I still hoped to glean some fresh facts in this field of inquiry, which might serve as stepping-stones for the further progress of those who might follow me.

CHAPTER II.

A REVIEW OF THE OPINIONS HELD ON THE CAUSES OF HAY-FEVER.

§ 30. In the last chapter I have mentioned incidentally that in its two principal phases hay-fever resembles common catarrh and ordinary asthma. Although this description is very partial and imperfect, it will suffice for our present purpose. When we come to consider the symptoms of the disorder in detail, I shall then be able to note their peculiarities, and to give to each its due significance.

In the present chapter I propose to pass under review the leading opinions which have been held on the causes of the ailment. We shall by this means have a better idea of their variations and peculiarities than would be had if they were introduced in a fragmentary manner in the course of remarks on other parts of the subject, and we shall to some extent have the ground mapped out which I have had to occupy in my experiments.

§ 31. Not only have the opinions which have been entertained on the causes been very varied, but, as I have before hinted, these have in some cases been very conflicting. The most opposite conditions have, by some writers and also patients, been thought to be capable of producing the disorder.

In some cases high temperature with dryness of the atmosphere have been held to be sufficient to produce the symptoms of hay-fever in persons who are liable to it. Some patients have thought that excess of moisture with high temperature has brought on the disorder in their cases. By some authors ozone is named as a possible exciting cause of the disease, and by others odours of various kinds, especially those given off by plants, have been accused of being the causes. In some cases common dust has been thought to have a considerable share in bringing on the disorder, whilst in a comparatively large number of instances the agent which has given the popular name to the malady has been taken to be the principal if not the only exciting cause. In an equally large number of instances, however, the pollen of grass, and other flowering plants, has been held to be the most active and efficient of all causes, but among these the pollen of grass is by some writers held to be the most powerful.

§ 32. Upon one point, however, all authors are agreed, viz., on the existence of some peculiarity of the constitution which predisposes to the disease. Whether this peculiarity should, however, be regarded as simply a local one, to be found in a particular vascular, or other, condition of the mucous membranes affected, or whether it is to be sought for in the periphery of the nerve, or in some part of the nerve tract supplying these membranes, or whether we must go to the sympathetic system, or to the larger nerve-centres, and seek there for the predisposing cause of the malady, is not yet decided. Curious and unaccountable as the predisposition seems to be, we shall, when we know more of its nature than we now do, probably find that, in the modes of its manifestation, and in the laws which govern these, it does not differ very widely from the peculiarities which give a proclivity to other and essentially different forms of disease.

§ 33. Bostock, who was the first writer who gave a full description of the ailment, believed that in his case it was not caused by the effluvium of grass or hay. He thought that heat had the greatest share of influence in producing the attacks. After the attention of the public had been drawn to the existence of the disease, probably by the publication of his first paper, the idea prevailed that it was caused by the effluvium of hay recently made. Bostock was desirous of testing the accuracy of this opinion, and made it the subject of study and close observation so that he might be able to determine the cause of the attacks in his own case.

In speaking of this part of the subject, after he had

carefully studied it and watched the effects of variations of temperature and other conditions; and especially after he had, as he thought, watched the effects which grass in flower, and also when turned into hay, had in producing the attacks, he says :—*

"I think myself fully warranted in asserting that, in my own case, the effluvium from hay has no connection with the disease. The observations will, I think, be sufficient to prove this position.

"In consequence of the benefit which I always experience from cool fresh air I made choice of Ramsgate as my residence during the summers of 1824, 1825, and 1826. The last two of these years will be long remembered for their excessive heat; but by procuring a house on the cliff exposed to the German Ocean, and commanding complete ventilation, by avoiding bodily exercise, and, indeed, seldom leaving the house until evening; during the year 1825 I nearly escaped the disease. In the year 1826 I have reason to believe that the disease was much mitigated by the comparative coolness of the situation, but still I had many decided and some severe paroxysms.

"Now it is well known that there is not an acre of meadow-ground in the whole of the Isle of Thanet, and in the year 1826, in consequence of the great drought, all the little patches of grass which may be supposed to exist on the road sides, or elsewhere, were completely burnt up.

"Nor is this all, during many of the hottest days the wind blew steadily from the south-east, so that the nearest land to windward of the house which I occupied was on the French coast a little to the north of Calais. Yet, during this time, whenever I relaxed my plan of discipline, and exposed myself to the sun's rays or by any means quickened the circulation, the symptoms recurred in full force.

"The last year, 1827, with the exception of a short period in July, was cold. I could not conveniently remove to any great distance from London, and spent the summer in Kew. This situation might have been chosen for the purpose of experiment, for almost the whole of that part of the country consists of hay-grass, which was cut whilst I

* *Medico-Chirurgical Transactions*, 1828, vol. xii, pp. 437—446.

was in the neighbourhood. In consequence of the coolness of the season I did not confine myself to the house, but walked out daily, occasionally in Kew Gardens, and was surrounded by many hundreds of acres of hay-grass, in all different states, yet except during the few hot days, when I suffered as usual, my complaint was in a much less degree than the average. But although I think the evidence, so far as respects myself, to be quite decisive, I acknowledge that I have received accounts from various quarters of individuals who have felt no doubt, that the complaint was brought on by the effluvium from hay, and was relieved or prevented by avoiding this effluvium. I will not venture to assert that this opinion is incorrect, but I believe that in most cases we may explain the facts more naturally by supposing that the patients, at the time when they conceived themselves to be inhaling the effluvium from hay, were also exposed to heated air or sunshine, or had been using bodily exercise. Experience, however, must decide the question, and when the subject is once fairly brought into view it will not be difficult to collect a sufficient number of facts to enable us to form an opinion."

There is, in these observations of Bostock's, an evident effort to ascertain by careful experiment the real cause of hay-fever. It is this honesty of purpose which has probably led subsequent writers to accept his conclusions without submitting them to a searching examination such as their importance demanded; and his statements have also probably given the cue to some authors who have written on the disease without having had any personal experience of it. How far these statements of Bostock's are borne out by the results of actual experiments I shall have occasion to notice further on.

§ 34. Gordon, who was a contemporary of Bostock's, took a different view of the cause of hay-fever. Whilst he recognized the circumstance that many cases were on record which showed that severe derangement of the function of respiration was sometimes " occasioned by the odour exhaled by aromatic pungent bodies," he thought there could be no doubt that hay-fever was caused by the " aroma emitted by the flowers of grass, particularly from those of the *Anthoxanthum odoratum.*"

He had been inclined to adopt this view by noticing that "whenever the patient remained closely shut up in a house, even though this was situated in the midst of the richest grass, he suffered considerably less than if he walked abroad into the fields; and if he removed from the country to the centre of a large town he was never at all affected; but the moment he came into or approached a meadow he immediately began to sneeze and returned home with wheezing and difficult respiration."

In summing up his observations Gordon says:—*

"I have said that the *Anthoxanthum odoratum* seems to be the principal exciting cause of hay-asthma, and I am induced to come to this conclusion—*first,* because this plant is one of the most strong-scented of the grasses; and *secondly,* because so soon as it begins to flower, and not until then, the asthma commences; as the flowers arrive at perfection the disease increases, and after they have died away I have remarked that patients could pass through the most luxuriant meadow with total impunity. The disease then should rather be denominated grass-asthma than hay-asthma, since hay seems incapable of producing it."

§ 35. Elliotson, who was also a contemporary of Bostock's, argues forcibly against the views entertained by the latter, and reviews his opinions at considerable length.† He, however, agrees with Bostock in believing that the disorder is not caused by hay, but, contrary to what the latter affirms, he believes it to "depend upon the flower of grass, and probably upon the pollen."

Elliotson also contends that this view of the case is supported by the circumstances that the disease does not usually appear "till the grass comes into flower; and as long as there is any flower remaining on the grass the disease continues."

In speaking of Bostock's account of his experience in the Isle of Thanet, when he suffered very little from the disease

* *London Medical Gazette,* vol. iv, 1829, pp. 266—269.
† *London Medical Gazette,* vol. viii, 1831, pp. 411—413.

and when the heat was so great that nearly all the grass was dried up, Elliotson remarks :—*

"I can conceive that a minute quantity of the emanations from the flower of grass is sufficient to produce it—so minute that you can be in few parts of the country at all, without the chance of its reaching you through the atmosphere, emanating from some grass or hay."

And again, in speaking of Bostock's experience whilst staying at Kew, he says :—†

"Dr. Bostock mentions, as another argument, that he was at Kew one summer where there was a great deal of grass growing, but he did not then have the affection severely. He mentions, however, that it was a cold season, and in a cold season you are aware that exhalations do not take place to anything like the extent that they do in hot seasons. That, I think, would account for the difference. But what makes me believe that it does depend upon the flower is, that a lady has lately given me an account of her own case, in which the symptoms appear and gradually increase as the grass comes, more and more, into flower, till at last they arrive at such an intensity that she is obliged to leave home and go to the sea-side, and she is always relieved by shutting herself up in a room."

Dr. Elliotson also mentions that he had heard a paper read at the Royal College of Physicians, on one occasion, where the patient described suffered from hay-fever, and was always seized with the symptoms of this disease whenever she approached a field of sweet-scented grass: In reference to this case he says :—

"I do not know what kind of grass produces hay-fever, but this would make it appear that it arises from an emanation, for whenever the lady approached a field of sweet-scented grass she was always seized in this way."

§ 36. Macculloch, who wrote in 1828, briefly refers to hay-fever as a possible form of intermittent ‡ He speaks of it as a well known disease, and as I have before stated, says

* *London Medical Gazette*, vol. viii, 1831, pp 411—413.
† Ibid.
‡ *An Essay on the Remittent and Intermittent Diseases*, by Dr John Macculloch, London, 1828, pp. 394—397.

"it is produced by hot-houses and green-houses, and in the public estimation particularly by hay fields." He does not, from the fact of hay-fever being a periodical catarrh, mean to say that it must be, therefore, a mode of intermittent disease, but he thinks, from the circumstance of its "having a quotidian period and being the produce of heat and vegetation, it at least presents features of analogy which render it worthy of being noticed in his work, and also of being more minutely studied; as far, at least, as we can investigate a disorder generally too trifling to attract much notice."

§ 37. A paper published by Dr. T. Wilkinson King* is chiefly remarkable for the manner in which the author mistakes the true character of hay-fever and for the way in which it helps to confuse, rather than to clear up, the subject in the mind of the reader. Dr. King had suffered from the disease, he says, for about fourteen years, and thought it worth while "to set down his own conclusions, together with an additional fact or two," so that he might "point to and confirm more general views of disease." The various causes of the local irritations as given in books Dr. King thinks are more curious than instructive, and, after noticing the various conditions which affect asthmatic patients favorably and unfavorably, he goes on to say:—

"The preceding and countless vagaries are to be accounted for by simple principles. (Vide a series of papers on "Angina," *Medical Gazette*, 1841.) We have to calculate that according to circumstances, a certain number of hours having elapsed after exposure (specific or general), eating or lying down, capillary excitement or distension is to be evinced by uneasiness, obstruction, and various forms and quantities of secretion. Beyond this, we believe very few of the phenomena of hay-fever or asthma will remain unresolved. The time at which the affections prevail is the time of diminishing our clothing.

"It seems to me, in the first place, not unreasonable to compare these affections with summer eruptions . . . . . . I think I have, at different times, experienced most of the

---

* "On Summer Asthma, Catarrhus Æstivus, or Hay-Fever: its Causes and Treatment," by T. Wilkinson King. *London Med. Gazette*, 1842—1843, vol. ii, pp. 671—675.

symptoms described by Dr. Bostock, *but not only in summer*. I am subject to slight attacks of dyspnœa, especially on lying down, attended by a very slight ropy and clear secretion in the trachea. . . . . I make very little doubt, also, that these same catarrhal disturbances of summer are of more frequent occurrence under a less distinct form, namely, that of aggravation of affections which, in some degree, the sufferer considers as habitual, and almost natural to him. One cannot travel without incurring ophthalmia, another asthma. Many suffer in particular localities or seem to require peculiar circumstances to secure tolerable ease. The above considerations, and my own experience, make me conclude that none of the affections are positively and necessarily confined to any season, or such a specific cause as hay or ipecacuanha."

This writer evidently confounds ordinary catarrh and asthma with hay-fever, and if he suffered at all from the latter disorder he was labouring under a mistake in supposing that it could come on at any time of the year independent of any specific influence such as he names. There is one point however which Dr. King notices in his remarks, in another part of his paper which I have not quoted, in which, although contrary to the opinion generally entertained, his observations will, I think, be found to be very correct, so far, at any rate, as regards hay-fever. In speaking of the structures affected in this disease, he says :—

"I make some exception to the conclusions of Dr. Bostock, that the air cells of the lungs are especially affected; and I prefer to set down the dyspnœa as the result of turgescence in the lining membranes of the air tubes."

So far as hay-asthma is concerned I hope to be able to show, further on, that this view of the case is more in accordance with facts than that which is generally held by the writers on hay-fever at the present time.

§ 38. Dr. G. T. Gream, who was also affected with the disorder, did not believe that it was owing to any strictly specific cause, and held that the farina of grass had "no more influence in causing the disease than that of any other flowers." He says :—

"The dust from beaten carpets, from the roads, and from

other sources, produces the same distressing symptoms." And he further remarks, " I am led to think that in the middle of summer, from the end of May to the end of July, at which time hay-fever generally ceases, a quantity of fine dust floats in the atmosphere, finer than any which is in the air at other seasons, increased, probably, by the farina of the mass of flowers at that period in bloom, but that during the later and earlier months, the more frequent rains, and the dews at night, prevent these particles from leaving the ground, and I have been induced to suppose that this reasoning is correct by finding that however distressing the symptoms have been during the day, they are all entirely removed by a shower of rain : the face becomes cool; the irritation of the nostrils and the eyes ceases, and does not return until the heated atmosphere has again evaporated the fallen rain.' *

Here, again, we shall find that although, in supporting his views, Dr. Gream is somewhat wanting in that exactness and precision which should characterise inquiries of this kind, he has hit upon one very important feature in the phenomena of hay-fever, namely, the influence which rain has in diminishing the intensity of the symptoms.

§ 39. Dr. Ramadge speaks of hay-asthma as a variety of ordinary asthma; but. in this form of the complaint, he regards the exciting cause as being more obvious than that of other forms of the disease, " inasmuch as we can refer to a sensible aterial object the presence of which is known to produce it, and the removal of which i - are to be followed by its subsidence." After detailing the symptoms of the disease and giving examples of it, Dr. Ramadge goes on to say :—

" When we take these facts into consideration we need not feel sceptical as to effluvia from the flowers of grass, the odour of the bean flower, &c , being the occasional cause of the variety of asthma of which we are now treating."†

---

* " On the use of *Nux Vomica* as a Remedy in Hay Fever." by Dr G. I Gream. *Lancet*, 1850, vol. i. pp 692—693.

† *Asthma, its Varieties and Complications, or Researches into the Pathology of Disordered Respiration; with Remarks on the Treatment Applicable to each Variety*, by F. H. Ramadge, M.D. London, 1847.

§ 40. Dr. Hastings, in referring to hay-fever, says:—
"The disease, in its severest form, is common in June about the period of hay-making, and there can be no doubt but that in some peculiarly constituted persons, an emanation from hay, the exact nature of which is unknown, occasions an attack of the disorder."*

§ 41. Dr. W. P. Kirkman seems, so far as I can learn, to have been the first patient who has tested, by an experiment upon himself, one of the supposed causes of hay-fever—the pollen of grass.† He tells us that a day or two before Christmas he noticed, in his hot-house for flowers, one single plant of the *Anthoxanthum odoratum* in blossom, loaded well with pollen. He thought it would be a capital opportunity for trying this particular grass, so he plucked it, rubbed the pollen with his hand and sniffed it up his nose; almost immediately it brought on sneezing, &c., and all the symptoms of hay-fever, which continued for an hour and then left him.

§ 42. Dr. (now Sir Thomas) Watson mentions this disorder in his lectures,‡ and quotes the testimony of Bostock, Gordon, and Elliotson. He also gives accounts of some interesting cases of hay-fever which have come under his own notice, but does not enter into any lengthened consideration of the causes of the disease. In his concluding remarks, however, after mentioning that the powder of *Ipecacuanha* produces similar symptoms to those of hay-fever in some persons, he says, "these effects of a powdered root and certain emanations from grass or hay lend weight to the hypothesis which ascribes the influenza to subtle vegetable matter floating in the atmosphere."

§ 43. Dr. Walshe, in speaking of hay-fever, says:

"A singular variety of naso-pulmonary catarrh, which has been supposed to follow the inhalation of the aroma of the sweet-smelling spring grass and hay (*Anthoxanthum odoratum*), is known under the name of hay-asthma, hay-

---

* *Treatise on Diseases of the Larynx and Trachea, &c.*, by John Hastings, M.D. Edin.

† Quoted from Dr. Phœbus' *Typische Frühsommer-Katarrh*, p. 137.

‡ *Lectures on the Principles and Practice of Physic*, by Dr. Thomas Watson. London, 1857, vol. ii, pp. 52—56.

fever, or summer catarrh. The complaint occurs only at the periods of hay-making, or when the odour of grass is powerful, and is of exceedingly rare occurrence. The susceptibility to these emanations, indeed, constitutes a very remarkable example of unalterable idiosyncracy. Persons who have once suffered invariably have a return of the disease, if exposed even in a slight degree to the specific cause. . . . . . . The most effectual means the habitual sufferer can command of preventing the attack, is by removing at the season to the sea-side, by getting out of the reach of the odours of grass and hay. But so exquisitely sensitive to such sensations are some individuals that a land wind, blowing for a few hours only, will bring on an attack even at the sea-shore. Once the complaint is established, total abstraction of the exciting cause will not put an immediate termination to the seizure. I have had a very precise narrative of a case in which the patient retained his symptoms during a passage across the Atlantic."*

§ 44. Dr. Hyde Salter, when treating of the annual periodicity of asthma,† remarks that asthma occurring once a year is almost always winter asthma, ... "There is, however," he says, "one kind of annual asthma that is not a winter asthma, but a summer asthma; and that is that curious disease called hay-fever or hay-asthma. This begins and ends with the hay-season, and varies in the time of the year, according as the hay season is early or late. As long as the grass is in flower it persists, with that it ceases. Its visits are, therefore, restricted to about a month or six weeks in the early summer. It is not constant throughout this time as one attack, but comes and goes with those other symptoms of irritation of the respiratory mucous membrane, of which it is a part. The neighbourhood of hay, bright, hot, dusty sunshine, a full meal, laughter, &c., suffice at any time to bring it on. It often affects a sort of diurnal rhythm, being generally worse at night. While this condition lasts the asthma is often so

---

* *A Practical Treatise on the Diseases of the Lungs, Heart, and Aorta*, by W. H. Walshe, M.D. London, 1854.

† *On Asthma: its Pathology and Treatment*, by Henry Hyde Salter, M.D., F.R.S. London 1859.

severe as to deprive the sufferer of sleep for nights together, and he leaves his bed in the morning, pallid, blear-eyed, and worn out. When the hay season is over every symptom vanishes, and for ten or eleven months the patient may calculate on a perfect immunity from even the slightest asthmatic sensation."

Amongst the examples which Dr. Salter gives are the narratives of two cases which are interesting as well as instructive. The patients each tell their own tale, and this they do, in each case, in a very clear and graphic manner.

§ 45. The first case is what we should call a typical case of hay-fever, or what Dr. Phœbus would say, was an example of the "whole disease;" that is to say, of both the catarrhal and asthmatic form of the disorder. This case is instructive in the way in which it shows us that the catarrhal form of the disease may set in and continue to attack the patient for some years, and afterwards be followed by the more troublesome phase of the malady in the shape of asthma.

In this case the patient tells us that the attacks first came on when he was about eight years of age, and in speaking of their commencement he says:—

"I well remember the first attack of those symptoms which, now more developed and more regular in their appearance, I recognise as my annual hay-fever torment. . . . . . I was at the play-work of haymaking with my young companions, surrounded by newly mown grass, when I was suddenly seized with all the eye and nose symptoms of hay-fever—profuse lachrymation, swelling of the conjunctivæ and lids, with intense ecchymosis, well nigh blinding me, and ceaseless sneezing.

"I recollect that I was taken into the house by my elder companions, and speedily recovered.

"It was, however, about the fifteenth year of my age before I was conscious of my annual infirmity—before I understood that at every early summer I was liable to sneezing fits if I ventured into the country; but from that time to the present this tendency has been abiding, has manifested itself every year, and has always governed my habits and residence during the month of June, and part of May and July. . . . . . I am now usually first attacked by sneezing and lachrymation about the middle of May, though this is much determined by the nature of the season; the warmer the weather, and the more advanced the vegetation, the earlier does my malady show itself. It usually lasts till the end of the first week in July (when it leaves me very suddenly), though this also is determined by the rapidity and shortness of the haymaking season; for in a hot, dry season, in which the hay is rapidly made and carried, my immunity from trouble occurs a week or ten days earlier."

§ 46. The second case shows that hay-fever came on after the patient had suffered from ordinary asthma for many years, or that it must have been an accompaniment of the latter disease, without the patient having been aware of it. In commencing to describe the hay-fever symptoms the patient says:

"It seems reasonable to suppose that I must have been liable to hay-fever, at the ordinary season, during the whole course of my life, but till within the last few years I was never aware of its presence, or of the existence of such a malady. From the frequency of my asthma, and common colds in early life, it is probable that the recurrence of asthma at a particular season, and the other symptoms of hay-fever, were overlooked; and that when I became less generally subject to asthma, the tendency to hay-fever remaining, that complaint more distinctly declared itself; or it may be that of late years I have become constitutionally liable to hay-fever—either more suspectible of the influence, whatever it may be, or have acquired a constitution capable of evolving its symptoms. . . . . . . I have suffered most from paroxysms whilst taking country walks, walking through grass meadows, and especially in one particular garden surrounded by fields. The prevalence of the influence in this locality is very remarkable, as there is nothing peculiar in the neighbouring soil or its products. I know one other locality where the influence is still more excessive; here there is an abundance of flowering grass and rushes, the region is flat, the soil marshy, and in the neighbourhood there is a great variety of indigenous vegetation. If the influence arises from the grass, it is not necessary it should be cut and dried, that is to say, the presence of hay is not essential."

§ 47. In the early part of the year 1859 Dr. Phœbus (Professor of Medicine at the University of Giessen), who had previously taken up the special study of hay-fever, sent out a circular, which was published in various medical journals in this country and on the continent. The object of the author, in sending out this circular, was to obtain contributions on the pathology and therapeutics of the disease, and to extend the knowledge of its literature. Information was also sought on the following subjects:

1st. On the geographical distribution of the disease.

2nd. On the ethnographical distribution of the malady (that is to say, as to whether it affected natives or foreigners most in countries where it prevails).

3rd. On the influence of sex in predisposing to attacks of the disorder.

4th. On the effect of social position and education in producing a liability to the malady, and on the frequency or non-frequency of its occurrence among the working classes.

5th. As to whether the persons predisposed to attacks of this disease are distinguished by any marked peculiarities which make this predisposition at once manifest; and, in such a case, whether any such escape the attacks at any time.

6th. Whether any difference, such as is named above, is to be found in members of the same family, where one of the family may be predisposed to attacks of hay-fever, and other members not predisposed.

7th. Whether it always occurs, in those who suffer from it, at one particular time of the year, or at various periods of the year.

In the preliminary remarks to the questions, of which only a summary is given above, Dr. Phœbus draws attention to the leading features of the disease, and particularly to the circumstance of its showing itself *exactly* with the first heats of summer. In this latter observation there is, if not a little tendency to prejudge the case, at least an evident leaning to the theory of causation which the learned author has since adopted. Of this I shall have more to say hereafter.

The circular of Dr. Phœbus called forth a number of responses, and resulted in the accumulation of a mass of very valuable information on the subject. Several medical men on the continent, as well as several in America and in this country, sent contributions to the various medical journals, and to Dr. Phœbus, in answer to the inquiries made in the circular.

§ 48. Dr. Cornaz, of Neuchatel, Switzerland, has published an interesting paper* on hay-fever, in which he records the histories of six cases with which he had become acquainted. After giving the particulars of these, the author discusses the question of nomenclature for this disease. On the whole he prefers the name "catarrh," because in all the cases which he describes there was coryza, accompanied by catarrhal symptoms. The author also prefers the denomination "de foin" (of hay) to that of "d'été" (of summer), and the reason given for this preference is, that in each of the six cases, the flower of grass seems to be the agent which brings on the attacks. At the same time, however, Dr. Cornaz affirms that hay, when being gathered, will bring on the disorder, although to a less degree than the flower of grass.

The last-mentioned of these terms (d'été) Dr. Cornaz thinks might, in some respects, be considered an appropriate name, inasmuch as it has the very important advantage of not appearing to prejudge the cause of the ailment; but this advantage is, to some extent, counterbalanced by the circumstance that the name "summer catarrh" (catarrh d'été) is given to a disease which often sets in before summer has fairly commenced. On the other hand it is admitted that the term "de foin" is also open to objection, inasmuch as it is applied to a disorder which is known to lessen in severity, if not altogether to disappear, when grass has been converted into hay; and also because it is well known that, in some cases at least, the pollen

---

* " De l'Existence du Catarrhe des foins en Suisse," *L'Echo Medicale*, No. 7 July, 1860.

of cereals has the same influence in bringing on the symptoms.

§ 49. Dr Longueville,* who wrote an account of his own case in answer to the inquiries of Dr. Phœbus, tells us that he suffered from attacks of ordinary asthma, and says he also found that proximity to hay was sure to bring on similar attacks, but he did not consider that in the symptoms which, in his own case, followed those attacks which were caused by hay, there was anything which would warrant the designation "fever."

§ 50. Dr. Labosse, of Nitry, writes an article† in reply to the observations of Dr. Longueville, and takes the latter somewhat sharply to task for his statement "that there is not anything which should be called 'fever' in the symptoms brought on by hay." The former gentleman says we may have the feverish symptoms well characterised in hay-asthma, and he believes that the attacks of asthma from which Dr. Longueville suffered were widely different, in their symptoms, from true hay-fever or hay-asthma. Dr. Labosse had seen three persons who were annually attacked by this disorder, and in each case the symptoms were cough, dyspnœa, coryza, and injection of the conjunctivæ; and these began to come on precisely at the period when the natural or artificial meadows were in blossom, lasted as long as the time of blossoming, and returned periodically, every year, in those individuals who were subject to the disease.

In these observations we have the influence of the period of blossoming clearly pointed out, and it seems that in the case of the patient (a farmer) whose symptoms are here given, the influence of heat had never been supposed by him to have much to do with the occurrence of the attacks. It is also especially worthy of notice that whenever the *saint-foin* (the herb with which he fed his sheep) had gone beyond the period of flowering, to the ripening of the seed, the patient could handle it without bringing on any unpleasant feelings, or any of the symptoms of hay-fever.

* Of France, but of what city or town I have not been able to ascertain.—C. H. B.

† "Nouvelle Observation de Catarrhe de Foin."—*L'Abeille Medicale*, August 20, 1860, p. 270.

§ 51. Dr. Laforgue, of Toulouse, in a paper which was also published in answer to the inquiries contained in the circular of Dr. Phœbus, gives an account of two cases of hay-fever which had come under his own notice.* In one of these cases the patient is said to have always enjoyed excellent health during the cold weather, with the exception of an occasional attack of coryza, which, however, was never attended with any difficulty of breathing, or any of the symptoms of asthma. As soon, however, as the warm weather set in, she always began to suffer from coryza, and after a short time her breathing would become impeded, and as long as the warm weather continued she suffered severely from both the catarrhal and asthmatic form of hay-fever; and, in spite of all the means used to prevent these attacks, or to moderate their severity when once developed, the malady returned regularly every summer.

Dr. Laforgue thought that in this case heat was the exciting cause, and in concluding his remarks on this patient, he says:—

"The great heat of the last summer strongly affected Mdlle. X—; beginning with coryza, the cold (rhumes) has become such intense spasmodic bronchitis, that the dyspnœa has for several times shown a threatening character. . . . . . . This observation, methinks, enters well into the category of the facts collected by Dr. Phœbus, of Giessen. It furnishes a good example of those catarrhal affections which, developed under the acting influence of heat, present all the symptomological characters of asthma."

§ 52. In an anonymous paper published in one of the French medical journals† the author of the article, in describing his own case, expresses a very decided opinion on the cause of the attacks. In speaking of the effects of heat he says:—

"The heat has no extraordinary effect upon me; I suffer from it as anybody else does, but I do not feel any symptoms which may remind me of hay-fever. The hay being

---

* "Observation de Catarrhe d' été," par M. le Docteur Laforgue de Toulouse. *L'Union Médicale*, No. 149. 17th December, 1859.

† "Un dernier mot sur la Fièvre de Foin," *L'Abeille Medicale*, May 21st, 1860.

safely stored away, my pocket-handkerchiefs remain undisturbed until the following year; they only serve me for wiping my forehead during the heat of summer. . . . . After the hay is gathered in, the heat or atmospheric changes do not bring on, afterwards, any attack of coryza. Having the head only very lightly covered, the heat, however excessive it may be, does not trouble me any more than it does other people. But when hay-making is going on, at a time when it is much less warm than in August, I suffer in the most severe manner.

" I do not believe in an atmospheric cause or coincidence in regard to hay-fever attacks. I have collected many proofs respecting the effect of hay on my head in different countries which I have visited."

§ 53. Dr. Phœbus, to whom we are indebted for bringing together and putting into an available form all that was known of hay-fever up to the time he wrote, has pursued the inquiry into the causes of the disease with a care and minuteness which is quite characteristic of the mode in which the German mind deals with obscure and little known subjects. No phase of this curious disorder has escaped his scrutiny, and such has been the result of his labours that we may say with justice that we owe to him the creation of a considerable portion of the literature of hay-fever.

This question of cause is confessedly one of the most difficult parts of the subject with which we have to deal, but whilst it is desirable that we should enter into every phase of it with the greatest care and circumspection, it is nevertheless true that the process of refinement and subdivision may be carried too far, and in our anxiety to get hold of and to examine minutely every possible cause of the disorder we may fail to recognise the true cause, and may spend our time in the examination of those things which have no relation whatever to the malady, and which a more simple and logical method of viewing would have put out of court altogether If we have any fault to find with the way in which Dr. Phœbus has done his work, it is in the circumstance of the over-refinement which characterises that work, and the want of a more rigid process of elimination in considering its causes. An example of this latter fault is to be found in the reference which has been made to ozone as a cause of hay-fever, by Dr. Phœbus. Although this substance has been supposed to be a possible cause of the malady, it is well known to all who have paid any attention to its treatment that no method of cure or prevention is more successful than that of sending the patient to the very spot where ozone is most abundant and most constantly to be found, namely, to the sea-shore.* The great amount of time and labour, however, which Professor Phœbus has expended upon the investigation of this disease entitles his opinions to be received with respectful attention. At the same time, however, the conclusions he has arrived at demand a careful examination, because as he has embraced a wider range of causes of the malady than other authors who had written before him, he has, as a consequence of this, increased in a corresponding ratio the possible sources of error; and more especially because subsequent writers seem to have been largely influenced by the views he holds.†

§ 54. Like all other writers, Dr. Phœbus makes predisposition to be the starting point of the disorder, but in what part of the system this predisposition has its seat he does not attempt to decide; and he thinks that between those who exhibit a liability to its attacks and those who are free from such liability, no well-marked line of separation exists. Almost all temperaments and all states of the system, from feeble to robust health, are to be found amongst hay-fever patients. Curiously enough, however, Dr. Phœbus suggests that the predisposition may not be present during the whole year, but may "repeat itself annually at the season of the attack," and that it may possibly be produced in some unknown manner by the

* Lest it may be thought that I have dismissed this part of the subject in a somewhat summary manner, I may here say that I have not neglected to make a short course of experiments with ozone which will, I think, show conclusively —if any proofs were needed—that this body has no unfavourable action on hay-fever patients; or, at least, that it does not produce any of the symptoms of hay-fever. It is, however, only right to say that I should not, for the reasons I have given above, have thought it needful to enter into any experiments with ozone if I had not had other investigations in hand respecting it.

† See his *Typische Frühsommer Katarrh.*

action of one or more of the exciting causes. He also thinks it possible that the disease may be present in a latent state before it first shows itself, and consequently there is no necessity for considering the first attack as the commencement of "the whole disorder." For the same reason we may imagine the disease to be present in a latent state during the intervals in which the patient is free from any visible signs of it; and it may also be further supposed that variations in the conditions of the separate organs may possibly be a cause of the attacks having a somewhat intermittent character—occurring on one day and not on another —during the season when the disease prevails.

These views imply a possibility of the predisposition having been in some cases essentially of a temporary nature, but this is believed to be warranted by the analogy which exists in other diseases of a nervous character; but, as the author (Dr. Phœbus) remarks, "in no other disease in so constant and logical a form as in hay-fever." One thing, however, is considered certain, namely, that when once a patient has had an attack, this leaves a condition of the system which, to a certainty, leads to others.

It will be seen that these opinions of the modes in which the predisposition may vary in its manifestations are somewhat complicated, and also a little conflicting, but as some of the facts I shall have to communicate have an important bearing upon the opinions here advanced, I shall not enter into any lengthened consideration of them at present.

§ 55. Circumstances of a geographical and ethnographical nature seem to have a considerable influence in determining the relative number of cases which may be met with in natives of different countries. In some countries the disease is never seen among the natives; in others it is very rare. In respect to the comparative frequency with which the disorder is met with in the different countries of Europe, England stands at the head of the list. Germany comes next; having less than half the number as compared with England. France, Belgium, Switzerland, Scotland, Italy, Russia, and Ireland, follow in the order in which they stand. North America is said to have very few cases occurring in it, but this will probably be found to be an error.

The disease is said by some to occur frequently in that country under the name of " rose cold " or " rose-fever." According to a table which Dr. Phœbus has prepared, those who are of Anglo-Saxon parentage form by far the largest proportion of the whole number affected, whilst those who stand next on the list are the most nearly related to the former ethnologically. Out of a total number of 152 patients whose parentage was ascertained, 81 were found to have been born of English parents (natives of England proper), whilst of the remainder, 36 were found to have been born of German parents, leaving only 35 whose parents were natives of other countries. It is a curious fact, too, that we have only one patient who was born of Irish parents; thus showing that race seems to have a more potent influence in producing a predisposition to the disease than mere geographical position.. But it will probably be found, when the geographical distribution of the disease comes to be more fully investigated, that a change may be produced which will somewhat alter the proportions here given, but not to such an extent as to affect the principle here enunciated.

§ 56. Professor Phœbus places the exciting causes under three heads : viz , 1st. Causes of each single attack. 2nd. Causes of exacerbations. 3rd. Causes of the variations of the groups and of other variations.*

It is with the first and second of these I shall have principally to deal, and if we succeed in demonstrating the cause of each single attack, in any one year, we shall have made some advance towards discovering the second cause named, and probably there will not be much difficulty in showing that the causes of each single attack and of the exacerbations are, with very rare exceptions one and the same.

The third cause is more complicated and will not be so easily cleared up until more research has been devoted to it than has yet been expended upon it ; indeed, in the present

---

* Dr. Phœbus has also divided the symptoms of the disease into groups, according to the part principally affected, viz. into Nose Group, Eye Group, Throat Group, Chest Group, &c.; of these divisions I shall have something to say further on.

state of our knowledge, it is almost waste of time to speculate on the *causes* of these differences. Our first effort in studying this and also other diseases, of a more complicated character, should be to get a knowledge of the nature of the primary exciting cause, and of all the modes in which it may affect the organs upon which it acts.

The *causes* of the mode in which the agent acts, and the reason why it sometimes acts upon one organ and sometimes upon another, may for ever remain hidden from us.

In considering the evidence which has been brought in favour of the various substances which have been already noticed as being the active agents in producing hay-fever, Dr. Phœbus draws attention to the fact that some authors and some patients accuse one agent and some another; but no one, he says, "has accused these agents *en masse;*" and, although some experiments have been tried with one or another of these, no one has yet pursued a systematic course of experiments which, on the one hand, would prove that the presence of any given noxious agent (or supposed exciting cause) was always followed by an attack of the disorder; and, on the other hand, that the absence of this same agent has always given complete freedom from the attacks. Another source of error, Dr. Phœbus thinks, lies in the circumstance that "as soon as one of these noxious agents has caused its effect, the symptoms of the intensity of the disorder have shown themselves immediately," and it has almost always been overlooked that the symptoms of "the stage of development" had already preceded these, and the patients have thus taken the more complete form of the disease for the beginning of it. "If people in future," he says, "will be more attentive and especially observe more than one patient carefully, the author does not doubt that the accusation against these noxious agents will, in greater part, fall to the ground."

§ 57. Whilst recognising the fact that the attacks of hay-fever occur during the time that the greatest number of the natural and artificial grasses are in bloom, and that the duration of the disease is synchronous with the period of flowering, Dr. Phœbus thinks that the proofs which some authors have brought have shown "that this or that noxious agent of the grasses is not the only cause of the access, obvious in all cases," and with regard to these he says:—

"Such proofs were formerly very desirable but have now lost much in value, for we now know that more than one of these noxious agents is accused, with apparently good reasons, whilst *the first heat of summer*, however, is a stronger cause than all the grass emanations put together." He then goes on to say:—" I have already shown that the supposition that the attack begins with the first heat of summer, and that its occurrence depends on the latter, is supported by numerous and important authorities far more than the assertions which give the following as the causes: A, the common grass blossom; B, the beginning of grass being generally in flower; C, any blossoming grass not in too small a quantity; D, the first blossom of the sweet-scented spring or vernal grass; E, the blossom of rye; F, hay; G, roses in bloom; H, pollen of all blossoms; I, dust in general."

In concluding his observations on this part of the subject Dr. Phœbus says:—

"From what is said in the preceding paragraphs, I think myself justified in drawing the following conclusions: 1st. Nobody has yet succeeded in showing with certainty the exciting causes of each single attack. 2nd. With probability the following circumstances (momenta) may be accepted as such causes: A, the first heat of summer (which, however, only acts in an indirect manner as an exciting cause); B, the longer days (which act, perhaps, through the stronger influence of light, or, perhaps, also through ozone); C, the same (or nearly the same) odours and different kinds of dust which we positively know as causes of exacerbations of the attacks. Amongst these hay and the blossom of rye have the greatest probability in their favour. 3rd. It may be *possible* that one of these causes is the only true one, and that the facts in regard to the other causes have been falsely understood. It is more probable, however, and the after access especially speaks in favour of the supposition, that all these influences act as exciting causes of the attacks.

"Some patients might be susceptible to only a part of these influences.

"I do not doubt that future and more accurate observations, especially comparisons of the phenomena of the disease with the meteorology and vegetable phenomena, will bring certainty instead of probability and possibility merely."

§ 58. The English medical authors, who have written on hay-fever since the work of Dr. Phœbus was published, have, to a considerable degree, followed his teaching and, with some modifications, have arrived at much the same conclusions with regard to the nature of the causes; but, in some cases, they have gone farther, and have, perhaps, expressed the opinions he holds in a much more decided manner than he himself has expressed them.

§ 59. Dr. Abbotts Smith, whose work* has passed through four editions, gives numerous cases in which the exciting cause of the attack seems to have been the emanations from grass and other flowering plants.

He also states "that strong light as well as great heat will induce or aggravate the symptoms," but he does not believe that the ozone theory of Dr. Phœbus is sufficient to account for the attacks, or the exacerbations of hay-fever.

Dr. Smith mentions that M. Vogel, many years since, ascertained that benzoic acid exists in two of the grasses, which, by some authors, are considered to be the most important agents in the production of hay-fever, namely, the *Anthoxanthum odoratum* and the *Holcus odoratus*, and he suggests the question "whether hay-fever may not, in some degree, especially when it arises in persons who are affected by the aroma of grass or hay, be attributed to the irritating effects of benzoic acid, which is liberated from the above-named grasses by the agency of summer heat."

In support of this idea he says, "it may be observed that the attacks of hay-fever are almost invariably worse during the continuance of hot, dry weather, while they generally assume a milder character in wet weather, or when the temperature is much reduced; at these latter periods the

---

* *On Hay-Fever, Hay-Asthma, or Summer Catarrh*, by Wm. Abbotts Smith, M.D. 4th edition. London, 1866.

sublimation of the benzoic acid, contained in the flowers, would be less than in hot weather."

Dr. Smith states that he has been informed by Messrs. Davy, Macmurdo & Co., manufacturing chemists, " that the inhalation of the vapour which incidentally escapes during the sublimation of benzoic acid, causes considerable irritation of the throat and violent paroxysms of sneezing and coughing."

One case is given by Dr. Smith, which he thinks " bears upon the fact that the smell of decomposing vegetable matter is sometimes the cause of this affection." The patient says " I was occupied in adding fresh water to some flowers in a vase in which the water had been standing several days, and was foul, and as I poured it away my annual visitor came on."

In reference to this case I have to remark that it is surprising how easily facts may be misunderstood and wrong inferences drawn from them. It was a similar incident which occurred to myself, some years ago, which first drew my attention to the real nature of the cause of the malady. Of this I shall have to speak further on.

Another case is given by Dr. Smith as an example of the effects of heat. The patient had resided for seven years at the sea-side and, from his experience whilst residing there, considered that his case quite agreed with that of Dr. Bostock, in not being dependent upon the smell of hay " but merely on the approach of really hot weather. This year (1865) " he says, " the disease first came on whilst I was on the sea yachting with a friend. It was a hot day in May, with the wind from the south-west, the nearest land to windward being nine miles distant. I felt myself, after some exertion in assisting to hoist the sails, suddenly seized with sneezing and I have had it ever since." (The date of the letter was June 13th.)

After noticing the causes spoken of by Dr. Phœbus, Dr. Smith says, "each of the principal causes just enumerated has, doubtless, much to do with the causation of summer catarrh; and, as in all other affections, sometimes one, sometimes another, cause may preponderate;" but he afterwards adds, " the majority of sufferers from this disorder attribute their illness to the presence of ripe grass or hay in their immediate neighbourhood."

§ 60. Dr. Pirrie* thinks that there are two distinct forms of the disease. He notices the circumstance that the emanations from ripe grass and some other plants, in flower, are recognised as the grand causes of both the catarrhal and the asthmatic form of the disease, but he says that cases have come under his own notice where the sufferers have attributed their indisposition " to solar heat and intensity of light" and his own observations lead " him to conclude that sufficient importance has not been attached to their opinions on this point." One form of the disorder Dr. Pirrie regards as spasmodic in character, exhibiting its effects on the mucous membranes of the respiratory tract, and as being caused by subtle volatile emanations from flowering plants acting upon the nervous filaments distributed to these membranes. In some cases, he thinks the disorder may also arise from irritation of the filaments of other nerves, or it may be caused by a " primarily tumid and swollen state of the lining membranes" (of the air-passages) such as heralds in attacks of measles or common catarrh. In the other form of the illness it is thought that the cause does not operate directly upon the mucous membranes, or upon the nervous filaments distributed to these, "but on certain nerve centres of the cerebro-spinal and sympathetic system."

In the first form of the disease, Dr. Pirrie says, a change of residence and the use of other remedial measures are mostly followed by speedy relief. In both forms of the illness we may have severe catarrhal and pectoral symptoms, but in the latter "the vascular relaxation and the associated nervous paresis are the results of the debilitating effects of great solar heat, assisted in many cases by intense light, on the cerebro-spinal and sympathetic systems, of certain peculiarly constituted people."

Dr. Pirrie gives cases which seem to favour the idea that in these the ailment was due to the action of solar heat and

* *On Hay-Asthma and the Affection termed Hay-Fever*, by Wm. Pirrie, M.D. London, 1867.

light. Into the consideration of these I shall not enter at present.

§ 61. Dr. George Moore, whose monograph* on hay-fever is the latest treatise with which I am acquainted, holds much the same opinions of the symptoms and causes of the disorder as those held by the two last writers I have mentioned. He, however, expresses his opinions in a little more decided manner than these writers have expressed theirs; or, to put it in a more definite form, everything, or almost everything in relation to this disorder is a settled thing. The causes are with him clear and definite, and the symptoms are placed before the reader in a precise and exact manner.

Like the writers above mentioned, Dr. Moore believes the disorder is, in some cases, caused by solar heat and light; in others by the effluvia from hay or by the emanations from other flowering plants and from those of decaying vegetable substances.

Dr. Moore quotes Dr. Bostock's case as an example of that form of the disease which is caused by great heat and strong light, and he tells us that, in these cases, "sea-voyaging, out of the reach of putrescent and other effluvia, affords no protection or exemption." He, however, does not give us the particulars of any cases of the disorder which he has himself had the opportunity of watching, or of which he has obtained the histories. It is to be hoped that in a future edition of his brochure Dr. Moore will be able to supply the details of cases with which he has become acquainted, and particularly of such as have any bearing upon the question of cause.

§ 62. Another supposed cause of hay-fever is alluded to by Dr. Gull in his Harveian oration delivered at the Royal College of Physicians, June 24th, 1870. It was stated by Helmholtz that vibriones had been found in the nasal mucus of patients suffering from this disease. In reference to this supposed action of vibriones Dr. Gull says :—

"No new fact bearing on the propagation of contagious disease has been reached by the recent investigations on

---

* *Hay-Fever, or Summer Catarrh: its Causes, Symptoms, Prevention, and Treatment,* by George Moore, M.D. London, 1870.

dust; nor can we infer the nature of summer catarrh because the nasal mucus, under such circumstances, and at no other time, was found peopled by vibriones, since decomposing mucus is always populous with this common race of infusoria."*

§ 63. I shall now give extracts from the history of cases I have myself seen or which I have had communicated to me. One of these patients I have had under my care annually, since the commencement of the disorder—four years ago; and another of the patients who has suffered for about twenty-four years I have had under observation for about eight years. The other patients named have not been under my care at any time.

§ 64. Patient 1.—A military officer who has spent some years in India. In answer to my inquiries in reference to his case he says:—

"I was in India for some years, and during that time I had no hay-fever whilst in the plains; but one season I took an excursion into the Himalaya Mountains, about the month of June, and I found that on many days when I was in parts of the hills, which from their elevation correspond with the heat and climate of England, and where crops were growing somewhat of the same nature as European cereals, I had violent attacks of hay-fever, although no grass was cut for hay-making and the grain crops were nearly ripe. The cultivation, however, was very scanty and partial—small patches levelled in the hills about the native villages—so that I was more inclined to attribute the attack to the temperature than to the cultivation. Long grass, however, was growing in places on the hills."

§ 65. Patient 2.—The wife of a military officer, residing in the South of England. In this case the patient says:—

"The attacks always begin some time in May and occasionally continue until September, but in London they have

---

* I have examined the nasal mucus frequently in the early stages of hay-fever, but have never seen any sign of vibriones or any other infusoria. I have frequently seen minute bodies having distinct molecular motion, but this motion is not so vigorous or so extensive as that of most of the infusoria. I shall be able to show further on that some of these molecules are probably derived from the atmosphere.—(C. H. B.)

ceased about the middle or end of August, and they certainly seem to follow the growth of the grass, but roses affect me so severely that if I gather them a very severe attack instantly supervenes, worse than from any other flower. The attacks are very severe in a hay-field during haymaking, and the illness does not seem to cease with the haymaking season, but the climax of suffering hitherto, has been from the middle of June to about the middle of July."

§ 66. Patient 3.—Sir ——, Bart., in speaking of the exciting causes of the attacks in his case, says :—

"The attacks generally begin about the 4th of June and cease about the second week in July. In wet weather I seldom or never suffer. The hotter the weather (particularly if there is no wind) the worse I am. I am quite certain that, in my case, hay-fever is caused by the minute particles which come from, not only grass but, flowers and trees of all sorts."

§ 67. Patient 4.—In this case the patient is a medical man holding the rank of Surgeon-Major in the British Army. Having spent many years in India and being well acquainted with the climate, his testimony is, on this account, very valuable. In answer to my inquiries about his experience of the disease in India and in England, he says :—

"I have suffered from hay-fever for about thirty-five years. I have had it both in India and in England. The period at which the attacks come on is not fixed, the date of the attack depending more on the grass ripening late or early than on any other circumstance. They always begin towards the end of the hay season when the grass is fully in flower, and cease slowly and gradually—not directly—on gathering in the grass. In India the attacks come on after the rains, about August or September.

"Changes of atmospheric temperature do not increase or decrease the severity of the symptoms; I have been attacked as severely in the cool climate of Simla as in the heat of the plains. At sea I have escaped the attacks, and also at some northern stations in India—at Kurrachee for instance."

§ 68. Patient 5.—A lady residing in one of the midland counties sends me the following particulars of her case :—

"I have suffered from hay-fever twelve or fourteen years. The attacks generally commence some time in May, but they come on earlier in a warm season than a cold one, and they are sure to come on with the first scent of spring flowers. May blossom, or a bean field in bloom, is as trying as a hay field, and the Elder flower is the worst of all. The attacks sometimes cease before the hay is all gathered in; a cool grey day restores to temporary health, whilst heat and sunshine cause great suffering, but the symptoms are less severe after rain unless the weather is very close."

§ 69. Patient 6.—A young lady, æt. 22, residing in a suburb of Manchester. In this case the disease first came on four years ago. As far as she could observe there had been no change in the constitutional tendencies or in the habits. Each year the attack has commenced at the time the grass has begun to come fully into flower, and as long as the patient has remained under the influence of the emanations from flowering grass the attacks have continued. Each year, however, since the disease commenced the patient has, a few days after the attack has shown itself, removed to the sea-side. On every occasion this change of locality has brought relief in a few hours, and in the course of twenty-four or thirty-six hours the patient has described herself to be, what she considered, almost well.

On one occasion Blackpool, on the Lancashire coast, was selected as a place of residence during the usual period of the attack. On two other occasions, I believe Llandudno in North Wales was the place resorted to.

§ 70. Patient 7.—A lady, æt. 53, sister to a clergyman of the Church of England. This patient has suffered from the disease for about twenty-four years. When the attacks first came on she resided near Sheffield, but during the last eight years she has resided near Manchester. As far as the patient can now remember she suffered from both the catarrhal and asthmatic form of the disease at the commencement, but of late years the asthmatic form of the complaint has been the most marked.

The attack generally begins, in a mild way, about the

latter end of May. This goes on increasing in severity up to the middle or latter end of June, and from this time up to the middle of July the symptoms are somewhat severe; they then gradually decline and by the time the second or third week in August has arrived she is free from the disease. The disorder has attained its maximum severity generally about the middle of July—sometimes earlier and occasionally later.

Although grass in flower appears to be the most frequent cause of the attacks the patient has thought that flowers having a strong odour have brought on the symptoms.

On one occasion, when on a visit to a relative who resided near Bradford, in Yorkshire, she was out walking in a meadow where grass in flower was being mown, about the latter end of the month of May. She had not proceeded far when an asthmatic attack came on and she found it necessary to leave the neighbourhood as soon as possible.

Atmospheric changes of temperature do not increase or decrease the severity of the symptoms. She has sometimes felt as well in the latter part of August, when the weather has been excessively hot, as she has been at any part of the year (so far as hay-fever is concerned). She has also often found that a room with the windows closed, and the heat greatly increased by this means, has been much less injurious than it has been when the windows have been opened and the room cooled.

Rain always mitigates the severity of the attacks.

§ 71. Patient 8 (the author's own case).—I have, as I have previously said, suffered from hay-fever for more than twenty years, but the exact time at which the disorder first commenced I cannot now remember. The attacks at first lasted only a few days, and then declined rapidly; and they seemed then, to me, to be in some way dependent upon the commencement of warm weather. For several of the earlier years the attacks came on about the middle or latter end of June, but I noticed that a cold season would delay the time for a week or ten days. Up to the present time the disease has only taken on the catarrhal form with me, but I have once or twice artificially brought on slight asthmatic attacks. From the circumstance of my noticing that the advent of the disorder seemed always to occur when the heat began to be such as warranted the designation "summer weather," and particularly from the fact that a walk into the country on a hot sunny day, whilst the attack of hay-fever was on me, was invariably attended by a great increase of the severity of the symptoms, I was inclined to regard heat as the principal cause of the disease. After hearing of Bostock's case I was still more inclined to take this view of the cause, but circumstances which occurred subsequently considerably altered my opinions.

In the year 1857 I had occasion to go down to the seaside* for a day or two. The hay had been nearly all gathered in in the neighbourhood of Manchester, and I was, as a consequence, just beginning to feel free from my usual summer illness. When I had got within the distance of six or eight miles from the sea shore, I felt that my old enemy was coming on again, and before three hours had elapsed I was suffering as severely as I had done during any part of the attack I was just recovering from. The disorder did not at all abate for the time I then remained (two days). The heat was certainly not greater than it had been in Manchester.† I returned home at the end of the time named, and was not a little surprised to find that, from the time I reached Manchester, my hay-fever rapidly disappeared.

In about five days I made another journey to the same part of the sea coast, and when about the same distance from the sea shore, that I was when the attacks came on on the former journey, I began again to have all the characteristic symptoms of hay-fever; but, strange to say, when I got to my journey's end these again quickly disappeared, and I was not troubled again during my stay of seven or eight days.

I was considerably puzzled with the very erratic manner in which the disease had come and gone after the usual

---

* Blackpool, on the Lancashire coast.

† I made memoranda of the heat at the time, but these I have unfortunately mislaid, and cannot now find them. I have, however, a distinct recollection of the fact that the heat was slightly less than it was on my leaving Manchester.

period of the attack was over; but in thinking the matter over, I remembered noticing that, at my first journey, the hay grass for some miles inland was uncut, and also that much of it was in flower. Another concurrence of circumstances also impressed me much at the time, and helped very greatly to alter my views with regard to the action of heat, namely, that during my first stay there was a land wind blowing, and that during my second stay the wind was from the sea nearly all the time, whilst the heat was somewhat in excess of what it had been during my first visit.

Another circumstance, which occurred in 1859, helped still further to cause me to doubt whether heat had any direct influence in producing the symptoms in my own case. A bunch of one of the grasses (I think it was the *Poa nemoralis*) had been gathered by one of my children and placed in a vase in one of the rooms at home which I seldom entered. I happened, however, to notice the vase in going into the room a few days after the grass had been placed there, and on disturbing it to examine it, a small cloud of pollen was detached and came in close proximity to my face. I commenced sneezing violently in the course of two or three minutes, and had what I considered a rather smart, though short, attack of my usual early summer disorder. As this grass flowers much earlier than the majority of the grasses cultivated for hay-making, and as there was little or no grass in flower in the meadows at the time, I was satisfied that the symptoms were due to the pollen which had escaped accidentally during the examination. From this time my experiments, I may say, commenced, and these have been carried on at intervals as opportunity has offered. With what result I must leave the reader to judge.

§ 72. The extracts I have just given of cases which have come more or less directly under my own notice, have been taken from the answers obtained to a set of questions, a copy of which was sent to each patient. These were framed so as to obtain as much information upon the causes of the disorder as it was possible to get without appearing to have a leaning to any theory which might bias the mind of the patient in giving the answers. To save repetition I have dispensed with the questions in each case and have thrown the answers into a connected form.

§ 73. In the foregoing quotations I have endeavoured fairly to represent every variety of opinion held on the causes of hay-fever, and although I have done this at some length, and consequently at the risk of being somewhat tedious, I have by no means exhausted the matter I had at hand.

§ 74. It will have been seen that, even before the time of Bostock, the popular idea was that hay or grass in flower was the exciting cause of this disease. Bostock, however, by his observations upon his own case, laid the foundation of the theory that heat was a much more active cause of the disorder than the emanations from grass or hay. His experiments seem, at first sight, to be tolerably conclusive, but when we come to examine them carefully, and to compare them with the observations of other patients and with the results of other carefully conducted experiments, we shall see that his reasoning was based upon the results of a mode of observation in which there were several sources of error which he did not discover.

With an acuteness which was quite characteristic, Elliotson not only took a comprehensive view of the phenomena of hay-fever, but at the same time did not fail to notice some of its important, though less prominent, features; and, as the reader will have seen, he pointed out some of the probable causes of fallacy in the conclusions which Bostock had arrived at. Although the opinions of the latter have had great weight with most of the authors who have studied the subject since his time, it may be said that opinions have been pretty equally divided between the two theories. Like many questions, however, which have remained in an unsettled state for a length of time, this question of the cause of hay-fever has given rise to speculation; and causes have been named which could only have been thought of in obedience to a strong impulse to catch at anything which seemed at all likely to have any share in the production of the disease, but which the simplest crucial experiment would have shown to have no such power as that which has been claimed for it. The question has in the last ten years so expanded itself that, from being, as it was at first, confined to the consideration of the two conditions named by Bostock, we have now at least half a dozen of these supposed causes presented for examination.

§ 75. When Dr. Phœbus took up the study of hay-fever, comparatively little had been done which could furnish sufficient data for accurate conclusions; and considering the state in which he found the subject, he has, perhaps, accomplished as much as any one man could have accomplished in the study of a disease in which there is so little chance of continued clinical observation. Not being himself a sufferer from the disorder, he had no opportunity of observing its peculiarities, or of making any experiments upon himself; and from the circumstance of the disorder being comparatively rare in Germany, he had, as he tells us, only the opportunity of observing one patient. If Dr. Phœbus had been himself the subject of hay-fever, and at the same time had had an opportunity of observing a greater number of patients, it is possible he might have arrived at somewhat different conclusions. As it is, however, he has become a warm advocate of Bostock's theory, but, unlike the latter, he claims for the *first heats of summer* a power which does not belong to the later heats of summer, and seems to infer that the former have some specific character which the latter do not possess. Of what this consists, however, he does not satisfactorily explain; nor, so far as I am aware, do any of the authors who have adopted the opinions of Dr. Phœbus on this point, make any successful attempt at explaining them.

§ 76. The necessity for believing that heat has different qualities at different times, and, as a consequence of this, has the power *per se* of effecting at one time of the year what it cannot accomplish at another, is one of the weakest points in the theory which claims that heat is one of the most efficient causes of this malady. Before we can accept this theory as the true one, it should be shown at what temperature, or between what ranges of temperature a patient, who is amenable to this influence of heat, will have the symptoms of the disease developed in him; and at what precise point he can depend upon being free from them. It should also be shown that at any time and in any place, where a patient happens to be who is known to be the subject of this form of hay-fever, when the temperature rises to the point indicated, an attack is sure to come on.*

On the other hand, in claiming for the agents named in the foregoing pages the power of producing the morbid conditions which characterise the disease, we should be equally exact in our requirements. It should not only be shown, in any individual case, that the attacks come on at a certain time of the year, when the substance, which is the supposed cause of the malady, is generated in the largest quantity, but it should be shown that at any time when a patient, who is presumed to be susceptible to the action of this substance, is brought in contact with it, it will to a certainty bring on the attacks. The cause of the malady should, in fact, be as capable of being proved to be so by repeated experiment as any chemical reaction is capable of being again and again demonstrated by the ordinary processes of chemical manipulation. In no case has this hitherto been done.

§ 77. In Dr. Smith's treatment of the subject, there is an evident wish to fall in as much as possible with the views of Dr. Phœbus, but at the same time to recognise and to give fair prominence to the views of English observers. There is, however, no attempt at recording anything more than what may be fitly termed fragmentary observations on the influence of heat, and of the other causes named.

Dr. Pirrie, as will have been seen from the quotations already given, has gone a step further, and has distinguished the attacks which are said to be caused by heat from those which are thought to be due to other and very different influences. He, however, does not give us the history of any case where the symptoms and the apparent cause have been observed, season after season, and where the dates and localities are given in the manner in which Bostock has given them.

In Dr. Moore's pamphlet we have the symptoms, causes, and treatment of the malady given in a most orderly and concise manner, but although the author has evidently

* Unless it can be shown that other causes are in operation which prevent the attack coming on.

devoted a great amount of attention to the disease, he does not give us the history of even a single case.

It is a larger amount of this kind of evidence which is most urgently needed to enable us to arrive at sound conclusions, and the absence or comparative smallness of which has hitherto constituted one of the great difficulties in the study of the disorder; whilst this has at the same time been an almost insuperable barrier to the attainment of correct notions of the value of remedies.

It was in order to supply my own mind with additional testimony of the kind I have alluded to above that the experiments, which will be described in a succeeding chapter, were commenced.

It would be unreasonable to suppose that the experience of one individual could furnish an amount of evidence large enough to permit us to hold the question of cause, in any disease, as being a settled point, but whilst I cannot claim to have determined this for all cases of hay-fever, I believe that in doing so for my own case I shall at least have shown the way in which this may be done in a very large majority, if not in all, of the cases of the same character; and I am convinced that the more closely we study the malady, the more we shall find that, to a much larger extent than has hitherto been supposed, it is unique in the nature of its causes and in its character also.

CHAPTER III.

EXPERIMENTS WITH THE PRESUMED CAUSES OF HAY-FEVER.

§ 78. The object aimed at in these experiments has been to single out the agent which I believed was, in my own case, the principal if not the only exciting cause of the disease ; but I have also wished to show the ground I have gone over, as well as to indicate the point I have arrived at, in the hope that some one else may be induced to take up a similar line of investigation, and thus assist in correcting or in strengthening the conclusions I have come to.

The plan adopted has been, where practicable, to make each of the supposed causes the subject of separate as well as of combined and repeated experiment, and by these means to endeavour to eliminate such as have no power to produce the symptoms of the disorder.

§ 79. In the early part of the course it was deemed absolutely necessary to make each experiment as distinct as possible, so as not to allow the results of one to interfere with those of another ; but in the latter part, when experience had been gained, and had shown that this rule need not be strictly adhered to, the experiments were permitted to follow each other more rapidly. This was often done where it was desirable to see what effect could be produced by the re-application of any particular substance when convalescence had not been fairly established after a former experiment.

Various circumstances which were to some extent unavoidable contributed to render the course of experimentation apparently somewhat irregular. The nature of some of the agents, combined with the accidental way in which these had to be obtained, made it often impossible to conduct the experiments in as systematic a manner as might have been wished. This irregularity, however, had one advantage, namely, that it has brought out the results of such observations in strong contrast with those which were made in a more regular manner and under more normal conditions.

§ 80. The agents which have been named as the exciting causes of hay-fever admit of several modes of classification. One of the best of these would be to place these agents in three categories, according as they are mechanical. chemical, or physiological in their action ; but here we are met with the difficulty of not being able to determine in all cases to which of the three classes an agent may belong, After close observation for a long period I am not able to decide which mode of action takes the lead in the case of the substance which I believe brings on the disease in my own case.

For practical purposes a very simple method of classification will perhaps answer better than a more elaborate one in enabling us to decide which are the exciting causes of the disorder. By this method of arrangement we place these causes in two divisions. In the first are included those substances which are more or less under the control of the operator, and which can be generated at pleasure or can be gathered and stored for future experiment. In the second division we place those agents which cannot be produced artificially and which are not capable of being controlled or altered in any way when generated naturally.

In the first division will be found *benzoic acid, coumarin* (the substance which gives the odour to newly-made hay), other *odours of various kinds, ozone, dust,* and *pollen.* In the second division we place *solar heat* and *light.*

§ 81. In respect to the facility with which we can conduct experiments with these two groups of agents there is a wide difference. In one case we can have these made under circumstances of our own choosing if not of our own creating ; but in the other we shall generally have to trust to observations merely, and these will often have to be made in the presence of disturbing elements which are difficult to detect, and frequently when detected are incapable of being set aside. These circumstances must exercise a considerable influence upon the manner of conducting the experiments, and upon the deductions we make from the phenomena observed, but at the same time need not prevent the conclusions we arrive at being sound and trustworthy.

The account of the experiments will be given in much the same order in which the agents are mentioned in the two classes into which they are divided, viz. :—

A. Experiments with *benzoic acid*.
B. Experiments with *coumarin*.
C. Experiments with *odours* of various kinds.
D. Experiments on the action of *ozone*.
E. Observations on the effects of *dust*.
F. Experiments with *pollen*.
G. Observations on the influence of *light* and *heat*.

A. *Experiments with Benzoic acid.*

§ 82. The experiments with this substance were tried in three different ways. 1st. By exposing the acid to evaporation, at ordinary temperatures, and inhaling the vapour.* 2nd. By applying a watery or spirituous solution of the acid to the mucous membrane of the nares. 3rd. By subliming the acid at high temperatures and inhaling the fumes.

§ 83. In the first form of the experiment the acid was spread thickly on glass plates containing a superficial area of one hundred square inches, these being carefully weighed before being exposed. The room in which the plates were placed was a small room about 15 feet by 12 feet, and was kept at a temperature varying from 65° to 75° Fahren.; the average being about 68°. The room was kept closed

---

* Seeing that *Benzoic acid* does not sublime at less than 293° Fahr., it seems useless to try experiments with it at ordinary temperatures; but as according to some authorities in chemistry it contains a small quantity of essential oil, which accompanies the acid during the sublimation, in the process of manufacture, it is not impossible that this oil may be given off at ordinary atmospheric temperatures, and that it may assist in producing the symptoms of hay-fever.

for ten hours at a time, and after being so closed I entered it and spent a couple of hours in it on three separate occasions, so as to breathe the vapour if any had been given off from the acid. No effect whatever was noticed, which could be fairly attributed to the presence of the acid in any of the three trials. The plates were weighed again at the conclusion of the experiments, and were found not to have diminished in weight after a lapse of forty-eight hours.

§ 84. In the second form of the experiment cold distilled water was saturated* with the acid. A small strip of lint steeped in this solution was applied to the mucous membrane of one nostril, and was kept in this position for an hour. Another solution was made by dissolving a quantity of the acid in hot distilled water.† This was applied to the nostril at a heat of 120° Fahren. in the same way as the one above had been applied. Another solution was made by adding two drachms of proof spirit to eight drachms of water, and dissolving in this mixture twenty grains of the acid. This also was applied to one nostril in the same manner.

In order to be able to distinguish the effect of the alcohol from that of the acid a mixture of proof spirit and water (minus the acid) was applied to the other nostril immediately after the conclusion of the last experiment. A slight burning sensation was felt in each nostril after the conclusion of the experiments, and the mucous membrane was found to be slightly reddened in each case, but there was no difference perceptible between the action of the mixture containing the acid and that which was composed of alcohol and water. These experiments were repeated several times, but no effect which in any degree resembled the phenomena of hay-fever was seen in any of the trials.

§ 85. In the third form of the experiment, ʒj of the acid was placed in a crucible, and was held over the flame of a Bunsen's burner, so as to cause the former to sublime more or less rapidly. At first the heat was applied gently, so as to allow the vapour of the acid to be only just per-

---

* Cold water takes up $\frac{1}{200}$th of its weight of the acid (Miller).
† Boiling water takes up $\frac{1}{2\frac{1}{2}}$th of its weight of the acid (Miller).

ceptible, but in later trials the heat was increased until it brought out dense fumes.

During the progress of these trials I was present, and, indeed, manipulating all the time, but had no sensations like those of hay-fever. I had some dryness of the throat, with a feeling of irritation about the larynx, and a slight disposition to cough; but these sensations were not so marked in my case as in the cases of other persons who were in the room with me during a part of the time the experiments were going on,* and who had never been the subjects of hay-fever. It is almost needless to say that in each of these trials I inhaled the vapour of the acid freely, taking especial care in some of the later experiments to inspire through the nostrils only.

§ 86. From the uniformly negative results of all these experiments with benzoic acid, when applied in the various ways I have described, I think I am warranted in concluding that it has no power to produce any of the symptoms of hay-fever in my case. Moreover, unless it can be shown that the acid exists, in the grasses in which it is found, in combination with some base or some other body which renders it much more volatile than it is in the uncombined form, on theoretical grounds only we are forced to the conclusion that it cannot possibly be a cause of hay-fever, since the heat which is required to volatilise it is beyond anything which exists naturally in the atmosphere in any part of the world.

B. *Experiments with Coumarin.*

§ 87. This substance is an odoriferous principle found in some of the grasses and in the plants of several of the other natural orders. It is one of those singular bodies which boil at high temperatures† only, and yet readily give off odorous

---

* In the case of one of those who was present with me the dense fumes of the acid brought on a slight cough with a feeling of suffocation, as if there was some little tendency to spasm of the glottis; but this passed rapidly off on going into the open air.

† Coumarin fuses at 122°, and boils at 518°, Fahr. (Miller).

vapours at ordinary atmospheric temperatures. Its formula is, according to the new notation, $C_9H_6O_2$. It is, as before stated, found in several of the grasses,* but it is most easily obtained from the Tonka bean † (*Coumarouma odorata*). A tincture made from the powdered bean in the proportion of one part, by weight, to ten parts of proof spirit gives a solution which has a strong odour of newly made hay.

The experiments with this substance were made, in my case, by placing ten drops of this tincture on a porcelain plate, and exposing this to evaporation in an apartment which was kept closed during the period of the experiment, except when I entered it or left it.

In about fifteen minutes after the tincture was exposed to the air the room was filled with a strong odour of newly made hay, and though the quantity of the solution was comparatively small, it was sufficient to cause the air of the room to be permeated with its characteristic odour for quite thirty-six hours. During this time I entered the apartment, and remained in it a couple of hours at a time several times, taking care now and then to move about, so as to inhale as vigorously as I should have done if I had been walking in the open air. Several other persons were present for different periods during the time named, but neither in their cases, nor yet in my own, was there any effect produced beyond the perception of the somewhat agreeable odour of newly made hay.

§ 88. Three such experiments as that described above were made upon myself in different years, and at different times in each year, but in no one of them was there the slightest approach to any of the symptoms of hay-fever.

Four experiments with this same substance were tried upon patients Nos. 6 and 7 (§§ 69—70). The first of these trials was made upon patient No. 6 in 1870. With the

---

* *Anthoxanthum odoratum, Holcus odoratus, Hierochloa borealis*, and one or two other grasses. It is also found in the *Myroxilon toluiferum, Melilotus cerulea, Melilotus officinalis*, and other species of *Melilotus* (*Legumenosæ*), also in the *Asperula odorata* (*Rubiaceæ*), in the *Prunus Mahaleb* (*Rosaceæ*) in the *Orchis fusca, Angrecum fragrans*, and *Nigritella alpina* (*Orchideæ*), and in the *Herniaria glabra* (*Portulaceæ*).

† By some German authors Coumarin has been called "Tonka camphor."

exceptions that the apartment was not kept closed during
the time the tincture was exposed, and the circumstance
that the patient did not remain quite so long at one
time in the room, the conditions were just the same as they
had been in my own case. Another experiment, with
exactly the same quantity of material, and under pretty
much the same conditions, was tried in the early part of this
year (1871). In both these cases there were several other
persons, who never suffered from hay-fever, in the room
during the whole time the tincture was exposed, but in no
case were there any unpleasant symptoms produced. The
patient, as well as several of the other persons present, very
quickly detected the characteristic odour of the coumarin;
but in no case were they aware of the object of the experiment, nor yet of the nature of the substance employed.

§ 89. Two experiments were also tried with patient No.
7, but under somewhat severe and more trying circumstances. In the first of these trials the quantity of tincture
exposed for evaporation was the same as in the other cases,
but in an hour after the experiment had been commenced
the quantity was doubled. The vessel containing the tincture was, during a good part of the time, not more than four
feet from the patient, so that the odour was very strong in
her immediate neighbourhood. An important circumstance
in this experiment was, that the patient remained in the same
room night and day during the whole time the experiment
was going on. In this case also the patient was not in the
least aware of the object of the experiment, nor of the
nature of the ordoriferous agent used. No symptoms which could fairly be attributed to the presence of the
coumarin were developed.

§ 90. The entire absence of results in this series of observations makes it absolutely certain that in these cases, as
well as in my own, coumarin has no power to produce any
of the symptoms of catarrhus æstivus.

c. *Experiments with odours of various kinds.*

§ 91. In addition to the trials made with coumarin, I
have also experimented upon the effects of many other

volatile bodies, amongst which I may mention *Paraffin oil, Camphor, Oleum terebinthinæ, Oleum menthæ piperitæ, Oleum juniperi, Oleum rosmarini, Oleum lavendulæ,* &c. I have also tested the odours given off by the flowers and herbs of wild and cultivated plants, such as the *Chamomilla matricaria, Rosa canina* and other species of roses, *Viola odorata, Lilium tigrinum, Lilium album, Cynoglossum,* and many other flowering plants which it would serve no purpose to enumerate here. I have also tried the odours given off by several of the fungi.

§ 29. The experiments with camphor were tried much in the same way as those with coumarin, as were also those with some of the volatile oils. In all cases they were made sufficiently exact to permit me to say decisively whether any of them had the power of producing the symptoms of hay-fever. The experiments with the vapour of the oil of turpentine were more severe and extensive than those with any of the other volatile bodies; but this was not because I believed it was more capable than the other bodies of generating the specific symptoms I was seeking for, but because the opportunity for testing it somewhat extensively, without any trouble or inconvenience to myself, came in my way. The necessary conditions were, in fact, ready made to my hand at any time when I chose to avail myself of them. I had the opportunity of visiting an establishment where a considerable quantity of copal varnish was used. In a room set apart for the purpose, from one to two thousand superficial square feet of varnished paper were often exposed at one time. Ordinarily copal varnish does not contain much oil of turpentine, but in this case it was the custom to add twenty or thirty per cent. of the oil in order to facilitate the working, and to help the drying. This, of course, was evaporated in the drying, and the atmosphere of the room was, as a consequence, highly charged with the vapour of the oil of turpentine. I have frequently entered the room, and have breathed the air for half an hour to an hour at a time. I have also taken the opportunity of doing this at the time I have been suffering from hay-fever, as well as when I have been quite free from it, but have not noticed any difference in the effect produced.

§ 93. The experiments with paraffin oil were tried under somewhat similar conditions to those last named, but were not so frequently repeated, nor yet could I say that the atmosphere of the room was so highly charged with the vapour of the oil as in the other case.

The volatile oils all produced head symptoms more or less severe in character, in some cases scarcely to be felt, but in other cases becoming rather unpleasant when long continued. The effects of the oil of turpentine were always the most marked, but this was probably owing to the fact that a much larger quantity of the vapour was inhaled than of any of the other substances. In no instance, however, were there any symptoms set up which in the least degree resembled those of hay-fever.

§ 94. The odour of the *Chamomilla matricaria* had a marked effect both upon myself and others. The plant had been gathered fresh in considerable quantity, and spread out in the room which we occupied as a dining room during one of our seaside visits, so that we inhaled the volatile principle given off pretty freely. Severe aching pain across the forehead, with nausea, dizziness, and pain at the epigastrium, were the principal symptoms, and these became so unpleasant on the second day after the plant had been placed in the room that I was glad to have it removed. There were, however, none of the symptoms of hay-fever produced.

§ 95. The inhalation of the odour of one of the microscopic fungi (*Chætomium*) also produced rather unpleasant symptoms with me, but these were not at all like the symptoms of hay-fever. The spores of another of the microscopic fungi (*Penicillium glaucum*) I have reason to believe will, when brought into contact with the respiratory mucous membrane, generate symptoms not unlike those of hay-fever in some respects, but differing materially in others—being much more like those of ordinary influenza.*

---

* I had noticed many years ago that the dust from straw sometimes brought on attacks of sneezing with me, and that this seemed to occur more frequently when we had had a long spell of wet weather. I determined to try what fungi could be generated on damp straw. For this purpose wheat straw, slightly moistened, was placed in a closed vessel, and was kept at a temperature of 100° Fahr. In about twenty-four hours a small quantity of white mycelium was seen; this increased slowly for three or four days, and in a short time

The sensations caused by these two agents were so unpleasant that I have never cared to reproduce them. In the case of the first-named fungus I inhaled the odour given off by the plant, on two occasions, in an experimental way. In the case of the second I was the subject of an involuntary experiment which gave me so much trouble and inconvenience that I have not wished, voluntarily, to subject myself to these again.

§ 96. The symptoms developed by the inhalation of some of the odours I have mentioned were sufficiently well-marked to make this a subject worthy of close investigation, but, as we have seen, it cannot be said that in any case the phenomena produced bore any resemblance to those of hay-fever. The action of the spores of *Penicillium* comes near to that of the exciting cause of this disease; but when the former comes to be thoroughly tested, I believe it will be found to produce symptoms of a much more acute and dangerous character.

From the results of these few experiments it is impossible to say whether the effects produced with the agents I have

after was followed by the appearance of minute greenish-black spots dotted here and there along the surface of the broken straw, apparently coming out more readily on the inner than on the outer surface. This, I found on examination, was the *Penicillium glaucum*. After a few days another crop of dark-coloured spots were seen, but these became almost jet black, and had quite a different contour. These I found to be the bristle mould (*Chætomium elatum*).

The spores of these two fungi were sown again separately on straw which had been placed in separate vessels after having been subjected to the action of boiling water for a short time. A separate crop of each fungus was thus obtained.

The *odour* of the *Penicillium* produced no perceptible effect upon me, but the odour of the *Chætomium* brought on nausea, faintness, and giddiness on two separate occasions. By inhaling the spores of the Penicillium, in the involuntary experiment of which I have spoken, a severe attack of hoarseness, going on to complete aphonia, was brought on. This lasted for a couple of days, and ended in a sharpish attack of bronchial catarrh, which almost unfitted me for duty for a day or two.

This experiment would seem to some extent to agree with the observations of Dr. Salisbury, of America, who states that he has seen the mycelium generated on damp straw produce many of the symptoms of measles among the troops engaged in the American war (the specific rash amongst other symptoms). (Vide *American Journal of the Medical Sciences*, July, 1862.)

mentioned are due to idiosyncrasy merely; or whether the liability to be affected by them is due to a constitutional condition which is pretty widely spread, is not at present easy to decide. In the case of the vapour of those bodies which are allied to the hydro-carbons, the liability to be acted upon by these will probably be very widely spread; but in the case of the spores of fungi, it is possible that the phenomena they exhibit may be restricted to comparatively few individuals; but, as I have said above, it is a subject which calls for much more careful and extensive investigation than it has yet received.

D. *Experiments on the action of Ozone.*

§ 97. It is to M. Schönbein, of Bâsle, that we are indebted for some of the most important and earliest researches on ozone. Since the publication of his memoir on ozone, in 1840, the subject has received a considerable amount of attention; but we have not as yet obtained a test which can at all times, and under all circumstances, be relied upon as an unfailing indication of its presence.

It is now generally believed that ozone is only an *allotropic* condition of oxygen, but Andrews and Tait, who have experimented very extensively with it, at one time thought it probable that it was a combination of oxygen and some other body.*

It is generated artificially in various ways, which I need not here stay to describe.

§ 98. M. Kosmann, of Strasbourg, made a number of experiments for the purpose of ascertaining the difference between the amount of ozone produced naturally in close proximity to growing plants, and away at a distance from any vegetation. From the results of these experiments he concludes that ozone is formed in greater abundance in the neighbourhood of growing plants than it is away from vegetation; but as his experiments were performed in the open air, without any apparatus to exclude the atmospheric ozone derived from other sources, his conclusions should be accepted with caution.

* Vide *Philosophical Transactions*, 1860.

§ 99. An interesting and important series of observations were made by the late Dr. Daubeny, of Oxford.* He found that, in addition to the other known modes in which ozone is generated, it is also produced by the action of sunlight on the green parts of growing plants.

By the use of an ingenious apparatus which he invented, the air was made to pass over growing plants, after the former had been deprived of any ozone which it had in it, and Dr. Daubeny found that these give off or generate ozone, when exposed to the action of sunlight, but not always in the same ratio.

§ 100. Professor Mantegazza, of Lombardy, has also shown, by his experimental researches on ozone, that this substance is generated by the oxidation of the essential oils of many plants. It was produced in large quantity from the essences of mint, turpentine, cloves, lavender, bergamot, anise, juniper, lemon, nutmegs, &c., when solar light and atmospheric oxygen were allowed to act upon them. It was also found that these substances have the power of ozonising a large amount of oxygen even when they are present in comparatively small quantities—so small, indeed, that in some cases where a vessel had been perfumed with an essence, and afterwards washed with alcohol and perfectly dried, it was found that if it retained the least trace of the odour of the essential oil with which it had been perfumed, it was still capable of developing ozone. Flowers which have a strong perfume were found to develope ozone in closed vessels, but those which were deficient in perfume developed it only in very small quantity or not at all. In most cases the direct rays of sunlight are required to generate ozone, but in some few diffused daylight is sufficient, but scarcely any of the essential oils will develop it in total darkness.

It is also very readily produced by the action of sulphuric acid on permanganate of potash, or peroxide of barium; and it is supposed that whenever oxygen is being disengaged from a base, ozone may be generated, but that this is not perceptible in all cases, inasmuch as it may be immediately

* Vide *Journal of the Chemical Society*, January, 1867, pp. 1—28.

taken up again by some other oxidizable substance present; but whatever is the source from which it is obtained it has much the same qualities.

§ 101. It is generally admitted that where there is a large amount of ozone in the atmosphere there—*cæteris paribus*—the best conditions for the enjoyment of health are to be had. Schönbein, however, found, during the course of his experiments, that when air highly charged with ozone was inhaled it brought on "a painful affection of the chest—a sort of asthma with a violent cough, which obliged him to discontinue, for a time, his investigations. Reflecting on this circumstance, he began to suspect that certain catarrhal disorders might be caused by atmospheric ozone. He got several physicians at Bâsle to compare their lists of catarrhal patients with his tables of atmosphero-ozonometric observations, and he and they were struck by the unusual number of catarrhal cases, on the days, or during the periods when M. Schönbein's papers (test papers) showed that ozone was unusually abundant in the air."*

From the results of these observations it would appear that ozone will, when present in considerable quantity, produce symptoms which have some resemblance to those of catarrhus æstivus.

§ 102. It will have been seen, from what I have said before (§ 53), that I do not conceive it to be possible, for ozone, in the quantity in which it is ordinarily found in the atmosphere, to bring on hay-fever. It would therefore seem to be inconsistent in me to be seeking for an effect which I believe cannot be produced. Whilst, however, I hold that we have abundant evidence to show that, in the quantity in which it is ordinarily met with, ozone will not produce hay-fever; we have little or no evidence to show that it may not do this when present in a larger quantity.

In this disorder, as in many others—and even in some of the so-called zymotic diseases—the *quantity* of the exciting cause may have almost as much influence in determining the occurrence of an attack as the *quality* has, and as I was investigating the effects of *all* the presumed causes of hay-fever, it seemed in this case also to be neces-

* Watson's *Principles and Practice of Physic*, 4th ed., pp. 47, 48.

sary to show by actual experiment that ozone has no such effect as that which it has been supposed to be capable of, even when present in what may be called maximum quantities, such as are often found on or near the sea.

§ 103. For the purpose of determining this question I instituted a series of experiments on the action of this subtle agent, and, on account of the important bearing the subject has upon the study of other diseases of the respiratory organs, I decided upon making an effort to ascertain the relative amount of ozone present at various points of the scale.*

The first experiments were tried at Grange, on the north-western shore of Morecambe Bay, Lancashire, during the latter end of August and beginning of September, 1865. Schönbein's scale and test papers were used, but I was at first not very successful with them. As I was merely testing for the effects of ozone upon the respiratory organs,

---

* The first test papers tried—made on Schönbein's method—were procured from one of the London makers. These yielded very unsatisfactory results. If half a dozen slips were exposed for a given time, and placed under exactly the same influences, I very rarely found that these slips were of the same tint at the termination of the experiment; and frequently it happened that no two of them would be alike. Another trial which I made with test paper which I prepared myself, according to Schönbein's method, was more satisfactory, but still was far from being as exact as was deemed to be necessary in experiments of this kind.

I do not know what may be the experience of meteorologists in this matter, but it would appear that that of the late Dr. Daubeny was in some respects similar to my own. In the concluding remarks in the paper to which I have already alluded he says—"I cannot rely upon different samples of either paper (Schönbein's or Moffat's) yielding, under the same circumstances, exactly similar results, and, therefore, am loath to confide in their indications as furnishing corresponding measurements."

By adopting a different method in preparing the test paper, I have obtained results which are much more uniform; and by constructing a scale on a given principle I have been able to make some approach to accuracy in determining the *relative* amount of ozone in the atmosphere, as shown at various points on the scale.

It would be out of place here to attempt to give the details of this method, but I hope to have the opportunity of doing so at another time and in another place; but I may here state that, according to the method I have used, I find that if the first perceptible effect on a slip of test paper be taken as *unit*, it will require more than 700 times the quantity of ozone to produce the highest effect on the scale.

and for the purpose of ascertaining the amount of ozone present, I did not pay much attention to barometrical indications, to hygrometric conditions, or to temperature.

I was quite free from any sign of hay-fever at the time.

As I have stated above, I was not then very successful in my attempts at ascertaining what *relation* the amount of ozone indicated by any point of the scale bore to that of any other point; but I think I was able to decide that at the highest point of Schönbein's scale (10°) it had not, in my case, the slightest perceptible effect upon the respiratory organs.

§ 104. The papers were exposed in a garden overhanging the shore and running down close to high-water mark, so that when the tide was in they were within about thirty yards of the water and fully fifteen yards from any building. In this situation the slips of test paper were fairly exposed to the full force of the sea breezes, but care was taken to shelter them from the direct rays of the sun.

Twelve experiments were tried on six different days, commencing on August 27th, and terminating on September 2nd. The papers were exposed for twelve hours at a time, viz., one set from 9 a.m. to 9 p.m., and another set from 9 p.m. to 9 a.m. the following morning. The periods were arranged in this manner in order to give an opportunity for my being in the open air during the greater part of one of the periods, and also for the purpose of comparing the amount of ozone registered during the day and the night.

I was present during the time of the experiments four days out of the six, and, except during meal times and sleeping hours, was pretty constantly in the open air and for the most part on the sea-shore close to the water's edge.

§ 105. The total quantity of ozone registered in the twelve experiments was 93° (Schönbein), the mean for twelve hours, being 7·75°. The highest point attained in this series of observations, in twelve hours, was 9°, and the lowest 6°, and from a comparison of the total quantity registered during the nights and the days it was found that there was scarcely any difference between the two. The total amount registered during the six days was 47°, and the total amount for the six nights was 46°.

The average amount of ozone present was comparatively large, especially if we take into account that the period of exposure was only twelve hours, but it must not, however, be supposed that because twelve hours gives a mean of 7·75, an exposure of twenty-four hours would give double that amount on a scale. My experiments have shown unmistakeably that it requires a vastly greater amount of ozone to increase the depth of the colour in a slip of iodised paper from 9° to 10°, than it does to change it from 1° to 2°; or, in other words, the higher we go in the scale the greater is the amount of ozone needed in moving from one degree to another. A similar set of experiments was made in the same spot in 1866, with much the same results.

§ 106. Another set of experiments was made at Southport, on the Lancashire coast, during the months of February and March, 1866. Here, however, I was not able to pursue the inquiry in so systematic a manner as at Grange, in consequence of my stay being much shorter at each visit, the longest period being not more than thirty-six hours. This was, however, generally sufficient for me to take an observation, and to enable me to note the effect, if any had been produced, upon me, when there was a large quantity of ozone present.

The amount was generally large when a sea breeze was blowing, and almost invariably low when a land wind prevailed. The highest point attained several times exceeded the highest degree (= 10°) on Schönbein's scale; and when this happened to be the case the wind was generally very strong.* On such occasions I found that ozone could be detected in close proximity to the backs of the houses facing the main street of the town. The farther I went inland the longer time did it take to produce a given effect on the test paper, and, as a matter of course, the nearer I approached to the sea the more rapid was the effect, providing no building intervened. The maximum effect was got at the end of the pier when the tide was coming in,

---

* It has often occurred to me that all ozone observations ought to be combined with the use of an anemometer, so as to be able to make due allowance for the varying rates of the wind.

and when a steady and tolerably strong breeze was blowing in from the sea.

§ 107. A few observations were also made at Blackpool during the latter part of October, 1869, but those which I consider to be the most valuable and the most conclusive were made at Filey Bay, on the coast of Yorkshire,* in the month of July, 1870. Here we have an expanse of sea from three to four hundred miles in a straight line, so that when a sea breeze is blowing, it has a long journey to make without touching land; consequently, whatever action the ocean may exercise in generating ozone, we may expect to have the full extent of this action exhibited here.

§ 108. On many days during my stay at Filey, the temperature was very high, so that the place and the season were favorable for observing the effect of heat as well as that of ozone; and, to use the words of Bostock, "the situation might have been chosen for the purpose of experiment" (which, indeed, it had been, so far as ascertaining the quantity and effects of ozone were concerned); for I also found the place favorable for determining other questions connected with the study of hay-fever, in relation to which a geographical position of a certain character, such as we find here, is absolutely needed before any approach can be made towards deciding these questions.

§ 109. A glance at the map of Yorkshire will show a narrow strip of headland † to the left of Filey Bay, which runs out to seaward, half a mile or so in length. This forms the northern boundary of the bay. At the extreme point of this headland is a low reef of rocks,‡ which are left high and dry when the tide is out, but which are for the most part covered with water when the tide is in, and especially at spring tides.

This was an excellent spot for experimentation, and was a favorite resort during my stay. I found here a large amount of ozone at all times—larger than at any other place

---

* About seven miles south of Scarborough. Apart from scientific considerations it is a pleasant and quiet spot to spend a summer holiday at, but for the archæologist, the geologist, or the botanist, it is a neighbourhood which is replete with matters of interest.

† "The Car Naze." ‡ "The Brig," or Bridge.

I had visited—but this was no doubt in part owing to the character and position of the spot selected for the experiments, and also in some measure to the force and direction of the wind during the time these were in progress. It several times happened that five or six hours' exposure would produce a depth of colour on the test papers equal to 7° (Schönbein), and in some cases, when the test was exposed for twenty-four hours, the colour was beyond the highest point (10°) in Schönbein's scale.

§ 110. One experiment was tried on the water, the test paper being a portion of the time three or four miles away from the shore. In two hours this gave a colour equal to 5°, but in a test paper exposed for the same time outside the house we occupied in one of the streets of the town (at right angles with the shore) the test only reached 3°, although the wind was blowing in from the sea all the time.

It is scarcely necessary to say that I was present during the time when many of the experiments were in progress, and frequently it happened that I was at the extreme point of the reef of rocks I have named for several hours at a time, so as to place myself fairly under the influence of the abundant supply of ozone found at this place.

§ 111. I have previously mentioned (§ 100) that ozone is formed by permitting sulphuric acid to act upon permanganate of potash (or, according to the modern nomenclature, potassium permanganate). For any experiment in which it is desirable to try the action of this body upon the respiratory organs, with some degree of certainty that we have no other disturbing influence present, this is one of the best means of generating it in a ready manner. A comparatively small quantity of the two agents named, if placed together in a jar or wide-necked glass bottle, will continue to give off ozone* for several hours, and at the commencement of the experiment will give off sufficient to colour a test-paper, placed over the mouth of the jar, up to 6° or 7° (Schönbein) in a couple of hours.

Several experiments were tried on the effect of ozone generated in this manner. The gas was inhaled as it formed, and the odour denoted that the quantity was, for

* And also oxygen in its ordinary state.

the space it occupied, much larger than in any other experiment I have ever tried, except, perhaps, where a current of electric fluid is thrown silently on the mucous membrane of the nostrils.*

Whilst describing these experiments, I have purposely refrained from giving the results in any case, for the reason that the same statement will serve for all.

From the details and the dates I have given the reader will have seen that the observations were made at all times of the year; in the autumn at Grange, when the hay season was quite over, and at a time when I scarcely ever had any of the symptoms of the disorder lingering about me; in the winter and spring at Southport, at a time of the year when I never remember the disease troubling me; and at Filey, in the middle of the summer, when I was still suffering a little from hay-fever. In not one of these trials with atmospheric ozone could I say that it had any unpleasant influence upon me. In the experiments made with that which was generated artificially the only effect produced was a slight sense of dryness in the throat, but there were not any symptoms of hay-fever set up, and I cannot say that at any time my experience corresponded with that of M. Schönbein. Perhaps it might be that in my case a much less quantity of ozone was inhaled than in M. Schönbein's; nevertheless, I am satisfied that I inhaled a larger quantity, at times, than is ever met with in the atmosphere in the same volume of air, and I think it is fair to conclude that it cannot at any time bring on this curious disorder with me.

§ 112. In addition to the experiments already detailed, two different sets of observations were made for me by patients who crossed the ocean to Australia in the latter part of 1866 and the early part of 1867.†

---

* This is easily done by having a sharply pointed wire connected with the prime conductor of an electrical machine. If the wire is insulated by cementing a piece of glass tubing over it, it may be held in the hand of the operator and the current of electricity will pass off silently, in the form of a luminous brush or cone, which has its apex at the point of the wire, whenever the machine is put in operation.

† Neither of these patients was affected with hay-fever, and the experiments cannot, therefore, have any direct bearing upon my own case; but as ozone has been so often mentioned as a possible cause of the disease, it seemed to be

The variations of temperature and other meteorological conditions were also noted, but as these have no direct bearing upon the subject we are considering, I shall not specially refer to them, but shall merely give such facts as relate to the quantity of ozone observed on each voyage, and to some of the circumstances which seemed to influence this. It will be well to observe here that the numbers will not always exactly agree with Schönbein's scale, as the test-paper was not made in the same way as his, or with the same proportions of the re-agents. Nevertheless, the numbers given will suffice to give a tolerably fair idea of the amount of ozone met with.

§ 113. The first patient went on board the vessel he sailed in on November 6th, 1866. He commenced his observations on the 20th Nov. Ninety-two observations were taken during the voyage. The test-papers were exposed for twelve hours at a time, viz. from 10 p.m. to 10 a.m. on the following day. The first observation was made on Nov. 20th, when the vessel was about one hundred miles from Lizard Point, and the last one on Feb. 20th, 1867, when off Cape Otway (Victoria). The total amount of ozone registered during the voyage was 572°, or a mean of 6·2173° for each twelve hours. The highest amount was 10°, and the lowest 3°. During the whole of the experiments ozone was never absent.

As in my own observations at Grange and elsewhere the time of exposure—twelve hours—should be taken into account in estimating the quantity of ozone met with. When this fact is borne in mind the figures show that the amount registered is comparatively large.*

---

an opportunity for trying what quantity is met with on the ocean, which ought not to be let pass without endeavouring to glean a little information, and thus to throw some fresh light on those very rare cases of the disease which are said to occur whilst the patients are on the sea.

* In comparing the amounts registered in different directions of the wind, some rather curious results were brought out; the two highest mean quantities obtained being with the wind at opposite points of the compass, viz. from S.S.E. and N.N.W. The observations made while the wind was blowing from the first-named quarter gave a mean of 8°, while those made whilst it was blowing from the opposite quarter gave a mean of 7·6°. With the wind from the N.W. the mean was 7·18° and whilst blowing from the S.E. it was 7°

§ 114. The second patient sailed from Plymouth on November 22nd, 1866. One hundred and twelve observations were taken, commencing on November 28th, 1866, and terminating on February 4th, 1867. The result of these experiments agrees in the main with those given above, and particularly in the circumstance that the quantity of ozone registered on damp or wet days was always much greater than on dry and fine days.* As in the other case, also, ozone was never found to be entirely absent.

§ 115. These experiments show pretty conclusively that if atmospheric ozone is a cause of hay-fever in any case, the disorder ought to show itself more or less frequently whenever the patient ventures near the sea, and as ozone seems to be always present on the open sea, the disease should never be absent whenever he is at a sufficient distance from land to be free from the influence of land breezes. We ought also to expect that if the disease is in any case produced by ozone it should vary in intensity with the rise or fall in the quantity of this agent. How far this is shown to be the case I shall, in reviewing the testimony of other authors, have to consider further on.

E. *Observations on the effects of dust.*

§ 116. In speaking of dust as a cause of hay-fever most

This sort of balancing or compensating action seemed also in some degree to hold good in the lower numbers; as, for instance, in those with the wind from the N.N.E. where the mean was 5·4°, whilst in those with the wind from S.S.W. it was 5·6°.

Whilst, however, the above results were brought out by comparing *sections* of the observations, a comparison of the whole experiments did not seem to show that in any one particular direction of the wind there was a larger amount of ozone present than in others.

* In the first set of experiments forty-five damp or wet days gave a total of 332·5°, whilst forty-seven dry days gave a total of 239·5°. During the first-named period the wind came from almost all points of the compass, with perhaps, on the whole, a slight bias to the south; whilst in the last-named period the wind was quite as variable, but came a little more from the north or north-east than from any other quarter.

For an interesting account of experiments on the relative amounts of ozone with various directions of the wind on land, I must refer my readers to the paper, by the late Dr. Daubeny, which I have already mentioned (*vide* note to § 99).

authors have used the designation "common dust." In the strict sense of the term, however, there is no such thing as common dust. A careful examination of the dust of any district will show that, in addition to those matters which may with propriety have the name "common" applied to them, it contains ingredients to which this cannot be applied, and the nature of which will to a large extent depend upon the season, upon the geological character of the district, and upon the nature of its botanical productions. The *number* as well as the *kind* of germs and other organic bodies found in the dust of any district will also largely depend upon the meteorological conditions which prevail in that district, so far as regards heat and moisture.

When I come to give an account of experiments tried for the purpose of obtaining information on this point I shall, I think, have abundant evidence to show that the statements made above are, for the most part, borne out by the results of a long course of observation. For the present I shall content myself with mentioning, and with offering one or two remarks on, the incident which first drew my attention specially to this phase of the question.

§ 117. I have several times noticed that dust could at certain times of the year produce some of the milder and less marked symptoms of hay-fever, but there was this peculiarity about these attacks, that generally they came on only during the time that hay-fever prevailed (and then as exacerbations) or immediately after the hay season was over, but never during winter or early spring.*

There was also another peculiarity which these attacks had, namely, that they were more fitful and more ephemeral, coming and going in a more irregular and transitory manner than the ordinary attacks of the disease ever do when they have once set in. At first I was considerably puzzled and was unable to account for the fitful appearance and departure of the symptoms. I also noticed that the attacks were more frequent whenever I had to pass through any dusty lane in the country, even when the hay had been all gathered in. I was consequently inclined to think, as

---

* With some exceptions, which I shall name hereafter.

Dr. Phœbus and others have since thought, that common dust was one of the causes of the disorder.

§ 118. In one of the earlier years of my attacks,* when I was just getting free from the disease, about the middle of July, I was out in the country and had to walk through a lane which was apparently not often used for the passage of vehicles. A carriage which passed me at a rapid rate raised a cloud of dust in which I was, for a time, completely enveloped and compelled to inhale pretty freely before I could get out of it. A very violent attack of sneezing immediately came on and continued at intervals for about an hour. As I had to pass over the same road on the following day, I determined to see if the same result would follow by disturbing the dust voluntarily. I found that I could bring on the symptoms in this way to the fullest degree of severity.

§ 119. The first examination of the dust under the microscope, made with that which had been scraped from the road, did not show anything very special. A second examination of the upper layer of dust† was more successful, and revealed to me the presence of bodies which I now easily recognise as the pollen grains of the grasses.

So far as I can now recollect, the weather during this season had been very favorable for the rapid growth and flowering of grass—first a few hours of rain, then a day of sunshine—and when this got to be nearly ready for cutting, and before the period of flowering was gone by, the weather had settled down so as to give three or four weeks without any rain.

§ 120. With the help of subsequent experience it is not

---

* As I had not at that time made up my mind to follow out any systematic course of observations on the subject, I made no notes of the occurrence, and cannot now remember the exact year.

† This was got by coating an ordinary microscopic slide with a film of glycerine, and by pressing this upon a layer of dust, which seemed not to have been previously disturbed for some days. A thin layer was in this way taken up. In the first examination the dust was placed on the slide in a dry state, but in the second it had a small additional quantity of glycerine added to it, and a glass cover placed over it. This was probably the principal cause of my getting so much better results in the second examination.

difficult to see why such a season as I have described should have given rise to a condition of things which would quite account for the symptoms from which I suffered, but it must be confessed that it is not easy to say why I had the attack more severely in this particular spot than I had in any other under similar circumstances. Perhaps if I had then been as well acquainted as I now am with all the various channels by which the *cause* may reach a patient, in out-of-the-way places and, as it were, at out-of-the-way times, I might have been able to explain the matter. At that time, however, I could only do as some writers on hay-fever have since done—speculate on the causes of the phenomena.

§ 121. Before I conclude my remarks on this part of the subject I must allude to one circumstance which has several times attracted my attention, and which will serve as one example among many others which might be given of the accidental and apparently causeless manner in which the symptoms of the disease may be developed. I allude to the fact that an attack of the malady has often followed a ride in a railway carriage even when the train has been going into a part of the country where the hay-making has been finished, and where, so far as could be seen, there could not be any possibility of the attacks being caused by hay or by grass in flower. I am now satisfied, however, that these attacks were generally brought on by getting into carriages which had come from places much more north than Manchester, and where the hay-making is much later. For a similar reason I think the disorder may be brought on earlier than usual by a patient travelling in and inhaling the dust in carriages which have come from parts of the country where the grass ripens earlier than it does in the part where the patient may live. That this is not a matter of mere speculation my own experience abundantly proves.

The incident I have related above along with the other circumstances alluded to caused me after some time to decide upon investigating the matter, but before I could do so satisfactorily it seemed necessary to make some experiments upon the action of pollen on the respiratory organs.

F. *Experiments with Pollen.*

§ 122. In the preceding pages I have shown that pollen has been named by many authors as one of the principal causes of hay-fever. No one, however, has, so far as I am aware, put this agent to the test by following out a systematic course of experiments with it.

In the early history of the disease the nature of its cause was enveloped in great obscurity, and those who suffered from it were few in number; it is not, therefore, surprising that greater success should not have attended the earlier efforts made to clear up this obscurity. But when we remember the great differences of opinion which have of late years been held on the causes of the malady, it strikes one as a most remarkable circumstance that authors and patients should have been content to go on theorising upon the cause of the disorder when a few comparatively easy experiments would, so far as pollen is concerned, have set the matter at rest in any individual case. It is, however, much easier to theorise than to try experiments, and especially when these would have to be tried on the theoriser's own person.

At the present time even, when so much more is known of the disorder than formerly, opinions are very much divided and also, in some cases, very loosely held. In some instances it is assumed that a disease which is as constant in its symptoms as almost any disease we might name owes its origin to causes which are as diverse in their nature as it is possible to bring together. It is, moreover, affirmed by some authors that at one time one of these dissimilar causes, and at another time another, may operate in producing an almost unvarying set of symptoms; or, in other words, that in this disease like effects are produced by unlike and totally different causes. I shall endeavour to show that these opinions are not supported by facts.

§ 123. In the experiments already detailed I have in most instances had to record only negative results. In the observations I am now about to describe we enter upon a very different course. Almost every experiment is followed by a greater or lesser amount of definite and unmistakeable effect which seems to point to pollen as the most powerful if not the only cause of the malady.

In investigating the action of pollen on the respiratory and other organs the questions which presented themselves were :—

1st. Can pollen produce the symptoms of hay-fever?

2nd. Does this property belong to all the pollens, or is it confined to the pollen of some one or more orders of plants? and, if so, to what natural orders does it belong?

3rd. To the pollen of which natural order, or of which species of this order, are the actual attacks of hay-fever, as they occur in early summer, due?

4th. Is this condition or property found in the dried as well as in the fresh pollen?

5th. To what special substance in pollen is this supposed action due?

Some of these questions can be answered more or less satisfactorily: others, there are which will still have to be considered *sub judice*.

§ 124. There are certain conditions which are required in the case of any agent which is to be accepted as the exciting cause of hay-fever. These are better fulfilled in the case of pollen than in any of the other agents, the action of which we have already considered.

In the first place, it should be shown that this agent, whatever it may be, will, when brought into contact with the respiratory mucous membrane, produce the symptoms of the disease to which it is supposed to give rise. In the second place, it should be shown that the disorder manifests itself whenever this agent begins to be produced in large quantity.* In the third place the attacks of the disease should lessen in severity as the production of this agent diminishes, and should be entirely absent during those parts of the year in which the latter is not generated.

* I have made "large quantity" a special condition because I shall have to show that the presence of a small quantity will not in some cases produce well-marked symptoms; but this term is, after all, only used in a relative sense.

Experiments with Pollen.

I shall as I proceed be able to show that these conditions are, in the case of pollen, very closely fulfilled.

§ 125. The first experiments were made with the pollen of the grasses, but the pollens of the plants belonging to thirty-five other natural orders were also tried. The experiments were made at all times of the year. In some cases the dried pollen was used after it had been kept some months, but for the most part this was used during the period in which the plants indigenous to this country were in flower, and whilst the pollen was fresh.*

This was tried in five different ways, viz. 1st, by applying it to the mucous membrane of the nares; 2nd, by inhaling it, and thus bringing it into contact with the

* Pollen from the following plants was tested during the course of experimentation, viz.:—*Aconitum* .... ? ; *Helleborus niger ; Ranunculus acris ; R. ficaria ; Anemone nemorosa ; Caltha palustris ; Aquilegia vulgaris* (Ranunculaceæ). *Papaver rhœas* (Papaveraceæ). *Fumaria capreolata* (Fumariaceæ). *Cardamine pratensis ; Nasturtium* .... ? ; *Cheiranthus cheiri* (Cruciferæ). *Viola tricolor ; V. odorata* (Violariæ). *Silene maritima ; Stellaria media ; Agrostemma githago* (Caryophylleæ). *Malva sylvestris* (Malvaceæ). *Hypericum perforatum* (Hypericineæ). *Geranium* .... ? (Geraniaceæ). *Ulex Europeus ; Cytisus scoparius* (Leguminoseæ). *Rubus fruticosus ; Rosa canina* (Rosaceæ). *Crategus oxycanthus ; Pyrus* .... ? (Pomaceæ). *Cucumis* .... ? (Cucurbitaceæ). *Conium maculatum ; Heracleum sphondylium* (Umbelliferæ). *Sambucus niger* (Caprifoliaceæ). *Scabiosa columbaria* (Dipsaceæ). *Arctium lappa ; Centaurea* .... ? ; *Tussilago farfara ; Senecio vulgaris ; Chamomilla matricaria ; Calendula officinalis* (Compositeæ). *Campanula rotundifolia ; C. hederacea* (Campanulaceæ). *Vinca minor* (Apocyneæ). *Convolvulus sepium* (Convolvulaceæ). *Cynoglossum officinale* (Boragineæ). *Solanum dulcamara ; Atropa belladonna ; Solanum tuberosum* (Solaneæ). *Veronica chamædrys ; Euphrasia officinalis ; Digitalis purpurea ; Linaria cymbalaria* (Scrophularineæ). *Mentha piperita* (Labiatæ). *Primula vulgaris* (Primulaceæ). *Plantago major ; P. lanceolata* (Plantagineæ). *Polygonum persicaria ; Rumex* .... ? (Polygonaceæ). *Euphorbium* .... ? (Euphorbiaceæ). *Betula alba ; Castanea vulgaris* (Amentaceæ). *Urtica urens* (Urticaceæ). *Arum maculatum* (Aroideæ). *Tulipa* .... ? (Liliaceæ). *Hyacinthus non-scriptus ; Allium ursinum* (Asphodeleæ). *Iris pseudacorus* (Irideæ). *Narcissus pseudo-narcissus* (Amaryllideæ). *Anthoxanthum odoratum ; Alopecurus pratensis ; Aira cæspitosa ; Poa pratensis ; P. nemoralis ; P. trivialis ; Lolium Italicum ; Triticum sativum ; Secale cereale ; Hordeum distichum ; Avena sativa* (Graminaceæ). *Eriophorum vaginatum* (Cyperaceæ). The pollen of a number of exotic flowering plants, the names of which I had no time to ascertain, was tried and yielded results much like the average of those given above.

mucous membrane of the larynx, trachea, and bronchial tubes; 3rd, by applying a decoction of the pollen to the conjunctiva; 4th, by applying the fresh pollen to the tongue, lips, and fauces; 5th, by inoculating the upper and lower limbs with the fresh moistened pollen.

§ 126. The incident related at § 71 seemed to indicate that the pollen of grass was at least one of the causes of hay-fever. Subsequent experiments confirmed the results of this accidental trial, and furnished an answer to the first question given above.

The pollen of a number of the grasses was first tried, and in every one of these trials this gave distinct and unmistakable evidence of its power to disturb the healthy action of the respiratory mucous membrane. When a small portion of pollen, just sufficient to tinge the tip of the finger yellow, was applied to the mucous membrane of the nares, some of the symptoms of hay-fever were invariably developed, the severity and continuance of which were dependent upon the quantity, and upon the number of times it was used.* In an experiment made with the pollen of the *Lolium Italicum*† the first sensation produced was that of a very slight degree of anæsthesia of the spot to which this had been applied. This was followed by a feeling of heat which gradually diffused itself over the whole cavity of the nostril, and was accompanied by a slight itching of the part. After some three or four minutes a discharge of serum came on, and continued at intervals for a couple of hours. The mucous membrane appeared to swell, and eventually became so tumid that the passage of air through the nostril was very much impeded. No sneezing occurred in this case, but this might partly be accounted for by the circumstance that the quantity of pollen applied was very small, and probably also by the fact that this was not fresh when applied.

* In the dried state 1700 pollen grains of *Lolium Italicum* were not heavy enough to depress the scale of a balance which turns easily with the $\frac{1}{700}$th of a grain, yet this small quantity produced a very perceptible effect when applied to the mucous membrane.

† A cultivated variety of *Lolium perènne*.

Experiments with Pollen.

§ 127. In another experiment tried with the pollen of the *Alopecurus pratensis* the lining membrane of one nostril was charged with the pollen by this being rubbed on with the point of the finger as far as this would reach. About one fiftieth of a grain was applied. Similar sensations to those described above came on, but showed themselves more rapidly than in the former case. In a few minutes a violent attack of sneezing came on; there was also a profuse discharge of serum, which continued for some hours, gradually diminishing towards the latter part of the time. In two hours after the experiment had commenced the mucous membrane had become so much swollen that no air could be drawn through the nostril in any attempt at inspiration.

§ 128. The pollen of *Secale cereale* (*Rye*) produced symptoms of a much more severe and lasting character than either of the grasses named above. In one experiment made with this pollen the sternutations were very strong and long-continued; the discharge from the nostrils was very copious, and produced more excoriation than in either of the other cases. The pollen was taken fresh from the growing plant, and applied on the spot, consequently I could make no attempt at ascertaining what was the exact quantity applied, but from the circumstance that fresh pollen is much more adhesive than it is when dried it is very probable that the quantity would be considerably larger than was usually applied.

The day on which the experiment was made was warm and moist—just such a day as would bring the pollen rapidly to maturity. A profuse coryza came on in less than a minute after the application. In thirty minutes the nostril was completely occluded, so that it was quite impossible to pass any air through it. During the day the sneezing and coryza kept up at intervals, and lasted for six or eight hours. During the night the nostril which had been closed became patent again once or twice, but curiously enough the nostril to which no pollen had been applied became almost entirely impervious to the passage of air,[*] and on each occasion violent attacks of sneezing came on.

[*] The cause of this phenomenon I shall be able to explain further on.

The experiments with *Rye* (Secale) were tried several times, and were always marked by decided symptoms varying in intensity according to the quantity of pollen used; having a milder character if this was used dry instead of fresh. The attack induced by three applications, at intervals of an hour, lasted twenty-four hours, and could even then be scarcely said to have cleared away. The discharge of the serum gradually altered by the latter becoming more inspissated, taking in this respect pretty much the same course as is seen in a case of ordinary catarrh, namely, by the discharge gradually changing to a puriform mucus, which, under the microscope, was seen to be much of the same character as that of the subsiding stage of ordinary catarrh.

§ 129. The action of the pollen of *Triticum* (Wheat) comes very near to that of the *Secale*, but is perhaps not quite so severe, nor does it develop its symptoms so rapidly. It is, however, quite as severe as that of any of the grasses, and seems to have a tendency to produce a more lasting impression than many of these.

In the case of the *Avena sativa* (Oat) the action seemed much the same as in some of the larger grasses. In two experiments which were tried with the pollen of this cereal, it was, as in the case of the *Secale*, applied whilst quite fresh. The symptoms were more severe and more rapidly developed than they are found to be when the plant is gathered and the pollen collected and dried before using.

Only one experiment was tried with the pollen of *Hordeum distichum* (Barley), consequently I am not able to speak so decidedly upon it as in the case of the other cereals and grasses. Nevertheless, its action was sufficiently well marked to show that it had, in common with the pollen of all the plants tried belonging to the order Graminaceæ, the property of disturbing the normal action of the respiratory mucous membrane in hay-fever patients.

In an experiment which was tried with the *infusion* of the pollen of the *Lolium Italicum* the action was very distinct so far as it went, but in this case there was no sneezing, and only a very small quantity of serum was discharged. The most marked effect produced was the tumefaction of the lining membrane of the nostril. This was slow in developing and equally slow in disappearing.

§ 130. The pollen *Lolium Italicum* was used with patient No. 6 on two occasions in a manner similar to that described above. In both experiments symptoms much the same as those produced in my own case were developed. There was sneezing, discharge of serum, and partial occlusion of the nostril.

One experiment was also tried on patient No. 7 with the pollen of *Alopecurus pratensis*. Profuse watery discharge from the nostril followed the application. There were also several attacks of sneezing in the course of a few hours, but in this case the occlusion of the nostril was not so marked as in my own.

In neither case was the patient aware of the nature of the substance used nor yet of the object of the experiment. In both instances the dried pollen was used. This was applied on one occasion early on in the year before the grasses were in bloom, and on the other in the early part of winter when few plants are in leaf.

The action of the pollen of the order Graminaceæ was on the whole very distinct and well marked. In some cases it was comparatively mild, and in other cases, as we have seen, somewhat severe.

§ 131. In the case of plants of some of the other natural orders the action was quite as well marked as in any of the grasses. The pollen of the *Corylus avellana*, for instance, developed its symptoms moderately rapidly. A small portion of this pollen was applied to the mucous membrane of one nostril in the usual manner. In ten minutes a violent fit of sneezing came on, and was quickly followed by a copious discharge of thin serum. There was a sensation of heat in the nostril, and there was also some oppression of the breathing, which in this case must have been caused by reflex action, as there was, so far as I could judge, no pollen inhaled. Why this should be the case with some pollens and not with others I am at present unable to say. I am, however, satisfied that asthmatic symptoms may be brought on as hay-asthma by reflex action. The mucous membrane of the nares was so much swollen in fifteen minutes after the pollen was applied that the air was with difficulty drawn through the nostril, and in thirty minutes the occlusion was complete.

The pollen of the common Tulip brought on a profuse discharge of serum, and produced great tumidity of the mucous membrane, but singularly enough there was no sneezing until the middle of the night, twelve hours after the experiment had commenced.

§ 132. One experiment was tried by using two different pollens for the two nostrils in as nearly the same quantity as possible. One nostril was charged with the pollen of the *Tilia media* (Linden tree), and the other with the pollen of the *Jasione* (Sheep's bit). The latter was the quickest in its action and also apparently the most powerful. There was first a sense of pressure in the nostril combined with slight itching; then swelling of the mucous membrane—or to speak more correctly of the submucous cellular tissue—and discharge of serous fluid. The latter was most profuse in the nostril to which the pollen of *Jasione* had been applied. The symptoms produced were much the same as those brought on by the use of the grass pollens, and the circumstance of both nostrils being affected at the same time did not seem to have any influence on the rapidity with which the symptoms disappeared. A walk in a park, where there were a great number of linden trees in bloom at the time, invariably brought on a smart attack of sneezing and coryza with me, and also seemed to have a tendency to produce more decided asthmatic phenomena than I have ever noticed when the grasses have been in flower.

§ 133. The inhalation of pollen, without permitting this to pass in any quantity through the nostril, generally brought on asthmatic symptoms, and in these cases only could I say that constitutional symptoms were developed. An example of this occurred accidentally in the month of March before any of the grasses were in flower.

In preparing the pollen of one of the Amentaceæ for the microscope a considerable quantity was accidentally inhaled before I was aware that it had been thrown off from the catkins so abundantly. A violent attack of sneezing came on in a few minutes, but this was not by any means so violent nor yet so persistent as I should have expected from the quantity of pollen which seemed to have been disengaged. Later on there was a moderately copious discharge of thin serum which kept up for some hours. After the sneezing and coryza had continued for a couple of hours the breathing became very difficult as if from constriction of the trachea or bronchial tubes, giving me just a slight experience of the misery those have to endure who suffer severely from the asthmatic form of hay-fever. In the course of five or six hours I began to have aching and a sense of weariness over the whole body, with pain in the head and spinal column. A very restless night was passed; the pulse rose from its usual number (68) to 100. Occasionally there was slight cough with expectoration of thin frothy sputum, and for twenty-four hours I felt as if passing through an unusually severe attack of influenza. During the succeeding night a violent perspiration set in, and as this proceeded I began to feel more easy. The pain in the head and the sense of weariness gradually abated, and at the end of the second day I was fit for duty again. In the early part of the attack, as I have mentioned above, there was expectoration of frothy sputum. This gradually changed to a thick puriform mucus, which was during the latter part of the time brought up for the most part by the mere effort of hawking.

§ 134. Another occurrence of a similar character took place whilst preparing some of the pollen of *Alopecurus pratensis* for the microscope. In this case the symptoms were similar to those given above, but not by any means so severe, and in addition to the symptoms detailed above partial loss of voice came on accompanied by a sense of irritation just behind the pomum adami.

One experiment of a similar kind was voluntarily tried with pollen of *Lolium Italicum*. A very small quantity was inhaled and was not allowed to pass through the nostrils in the process. No constitutional symptoms were developed.

The only symptoms were difficulty of breathing, as if from narrowing of the bronchial tubes, with slight cough and expectoration of frothy sputum. Probably the mildness of the attack was due to the smallness of the quantity of pollen inhaled.* The suffering and inconvenience caused by the former experiment prevented me from carrying this latter to such an extent as to run the risk of producing as much disturbance as in the former case; it was, however, carried sufficiently far to show that the possibility of inducing the most violent asthmatic symptoms was only a question of quantity.†

§ 135. With the view of ascertaining what would be the effect of a watery and spirituous extract of pollen when applied to the nostril an infusion of that of the *Lilium tigrinum* was made. The infusion was filtered, and proof spirit was added to the residuum, and this was again filtered after macerating for a few days. The two filtrates were evaporated to a syrupy consistence and mixed together. A portion of this mixture was applied to the lining membrane of the nostril in the same manner as the pollen had been applied. No effect which could be attributed to the application followed. The pollen of *Lilium* is not very active when applied fresh, but still it is sufficiently so to show that it possesses the property of deranging the action of the mucous membrane of the air-passages.

§ 136. A decoction of the pollen of *Gladiolus* was made by boiling a portion of this with one hundred times its weight of distilled water. One drop of this liquid was placed in contact with the conjunctiva of the right eye. The effect was almost instantaneous. The first sensation was that of intense burning and smarting, coupled with a feeling such as might be imagined to be caused by fine sand being blown into the eye. The photophobia was so severe that for some minutes the eye could not be opened for more than a single second at a time. In about thirty seconds the capillary

* Whether the constitutional symptoms in the first experiment were caused by the pollen I am not at present prepared to say, but I have no reason to doubt that they were.

† Probably also to some extent a question of *kind* of pollen.

vessels of the conjunctiva were seen to be greatly distended. With the aid of a lens the larger vessels of the conjunctiva could be seen to be raised above the surface. Movement of the eyeball gave great pain, just as is felt when dust has been blown into the eye. In six minutes the conjunctiva had become quite œdematous, but showed its closer attachment as far as the outer margin of the cornea. The œdema increased until very severe chemosis was set up. The eyelids also became much swollen. In two hours after the fluid had been applied the smarting and burning had much abated, and the congestion of the conjunctival vessels had considerably lessened, but the chemosis remained and was even more marked than it had been an hour before. There was a moderately copious discharge of fluid from the eye and also some little from the nostril. In six hours the eye still felt uneasy, but there was very little pain on moving the eyeball, although the vessels of the conjunctiva were still injected. The chemosis still remained as severe as before. In eighteen hours there was scarcely any congestion of the vessels remaining, but the chemosis was still very distinct. In thirty-two hours all traces of the derangement had disappeared. During the course of this experiment no effect was produced on the sclerotic coat of the eyeball, nor yet, so far as could be seen or felt, on the deeper structures. The action seemed to expend itself upon the conjunctiva and upon the cellular tissue of the eyelids.

§ 137. One grain of the pollen of *Alopecurus pratensis* was applied to the fauces for the purpose of ascertaining if it would have any effect upon the tonsils and upon the mucous membrane of the mouth and fauces. Slight itching came on in the course of a few minutes, and in half an hour the mucous membrane of the fauces was seen to be somewhat congested, but this was more seen in the engorgement of the larger capillaries than in a diffused redness. The itching was quickly followed by a sensation as if some hard angular bodies stuck in the throat. There was also a feeling of constriction about the fauces, although there was no swelling perceptible on examining the throat. I am, however, convinced from subsequent experience that the sense of constriction was caused by œdema of the submucous cellular tissue of the pharynx. The symptoms remained stationary for two or three hours and then gradually diminished.

§ 138. Whilst I was still suffering from my usual attack of hay-fever, during the summer of 1865,[*] as much pollen as could be obtained from two anthers of the *Lolium Italicum* was applied to the centre of the anterior surface of one forearm after the skin had been abraded as in the ordinary mode of vaccinating. A space of about a quarter of an inch was abraded, and to this the quantity of pollen named was applied after being placed on a piece of wet lint the size of the abrasion. This was covered with a piece of thin gutta percha, and the whole was held in position by a strip of adhesive plaster. The centre of the other forearm was treated in exactly the same manner save and except that no pollen was applied to it. The scratching with the lancet raised a wheal such as is seen in urticaria or in stinging with nettles. In a few minutes after the pollen had been applied the abraded spot began to itch intensely; the parts immediately around the abrasion began to swell, but this was not apparently due to any action on the *cutis vera*. The swelling seemed to be entirely due to effusion into the subcutaneous cellular tissue. There was no heat or redness more than what had been caused by the abrasion, and these were much the same on each arm. Although the swelling had the appearance of œdema, it located itself at first exactly around the abrasion to which the pollen had been applied, and gradually spread from this point and formed a flattened tumour, which had its centre at the abraded spot. There was no tenderness, and any part of the swelling was easily made to pit on pressure. The wheal caused by the lancet did not increase much in size after the pollen was applied. The tumour increased in size until it measured two and a half inches in length, by one inch and a half in breadth, and was raised above the ordinary level of the surface nearly three quarters of an inch.

[*] July 13th.

No pain was felt in the limb, nor was there any heat or redness present at any time, beyond the very slight amount to which the abrading of the cuticle gave rise. The swelling attained its maximum in six hours, and then remained stationary for other eight hours; after this it gradually subsided, and in forty-eight hours it had entirely disappeared. The arm to which no pollen had been applied did not exhibit any sign of swelling or irritation.

§ 139. In the latter part of September in the same year another experiment of a similar character was tried. Much the same effect as was seen in the former one followed, but the swelling was not so great, and subsided more readily.

In the following year the experiment was repeated by applying the pollen to the integument covering the centre of the right tibia. This spot was chosen because we have here only skin and cellular tissue, with a hard unyielding surface of bone behind these; consequently, whatever increase there is in the bulk of the part operated on it must declare itself more distinctly and more exactly than it is possible for it to do when there are soft structures underlying it. The same conditions were observed as in the experiment described above. When the pollen had been applied for a few minutes, the same intense itching of the part came on, as in the former case, but owing probably to the circumstance of the pollen being larger in quantity, this was more severe, and longer continued.

In about fifteen minutes after the experiment commenced the limb began to swell, and gradually increased in size, until the tumour measured four inches in length by two inches in width, whilst the centre was raised quite three quarters of an inch above the surface of the bone. The increase in the size of the tumour was much slower than in the other cases named. The swelling attained its maximum in about twelve hours, after which it remained stationary for other twelve or fourteen hours. At the end of four days the limb had assumed its usual size and form, the derangement having entirely passed away. During the time the tumour had somewhat changed its location, as if the fluid contained in the subcutaneous cellular tissue had gravitated; the portion of the swelling which disappeared last being quite an inch below the spot where the pollen had been applied. There was neither pain, heat, nor redness present during the whole time.

§ 140. The examples of the action of pollen given above have been selected from a large number. These give a fair idea of the nature and extent of this action. In most cases the experiments were repeated several times, and in some instances, where the details were not noted down at the time, the action was quite as severe as in those I have cited.

Extending as they do over a good number of years, the trials must have been made in very varied physical and mental conditions, even within the limits of health; but some of the experiments have been made when the system has been in a state bordering upon, if not actually suffering from, disease. I have not found, so far as I have noticed, that these varying conditions have had any influence in increasing or diminishing the intensity of the symptoms produced. It is, however, only right to say that my attention has not been specially directed to this point.

§ 141. With some rare exceptions, the action of the pollen of the plants named in the list given was sufficiently perceptible to show that this action was in some degree common to all. The intensity of the symptoms, however, varied in using the pollen of different plants, and also in that from the same plant at different times. There seemed, in fact, to be some circumstances which had a controlling or modifying influence upon the production, as well as upon the activity of pollen. Probably some of these modifying influences consist in those subtle atmospheric conditions, of the nature of which we are at present profoundly ignorant.

There are, however, some circumstances which exercise an important influence, and with whose nature we are tolerably well acquainted. One of these is temperature. A high temperature is in itself favorable to the generation of pollen, but a high temperature with severe drought will, in the case of the grasses, check their growth, and thus prevent the formation of pollen. In proportion as temperature and moisture are suitably combined, so will be the production of pollen, but where these happen to be unusually favorable, we may have the grass arriving at maturity rapidly, and as a consequence this may be quickly cut and converted into hay and housed. Under such circumstances, hay-fever patients may have a short season of attack, but the symptoms may be very severe whilst they last.

§ 142. Low temperature operates in quite another manner with the majority of the grasses. Growth may go on moderately well with a comparatively low temperature, especially in *some* of the grasses, but a temperature below a certain point will not permit the flowering process to go on in a normal manner. Not only will the quantity of pollen thrown off by a given number of plants be lessened, but that which is generated will have much less vigour than it has in favorable seasons. In the same manner pollen obtained from plants which have flowered prematurely does not seem to possess the same activity as that which is generated later. The pollen of *Bellis perennis* (common daisy) gathered during the earliest period of flowering, in the month of March, did not seem to have the same power as that which was gathered in the middle of summer, although this plant blooms from early spring to autumn.

Some of the cereals, however, will arrive at maturity, and maintain a vigorous and healthy condition during their period of growth, with a much drier state of the atmosphere and soil than is borne by many of the grasses. It is well known that wheat will thrive and do well with much less moisture than the grasses need. Thus it happens that in cold and wet summers hay-fever patients will suffer much less than in other and better seasons; whilst in a very hot summer, with continued drought, patients may almost escape the disease, even if they reside in a part of the country where hay-grass is largely cultivated. But when the cereals come to be in flower they may suffer very severely for a time. I think it was in this way that the attacks which Bostock had in the Isle of Thanet might be accounted for, and the mistake he made was in supposing that grass in flower was the only thing, besides heat, which could bring on the disorder.

Overgrown pollen also seems not to be as active as that which is fresher and younger. The pollen of *Atropa belladonna* (deadly nightshade) showed very little activity when gathered whilst the plant was in fruit, and when only a few half faded flowers were found on it. From the fact, however, that the pollens of *Solanum dulcamara* and *Solanum tuberosum* have only a mild action, it is probable that the pollen of *Belladonna* will not be found very active even when gathered at the height of its flowering season. This, however, cannot be considered a settled point; but certain it is that in some cases pollen is not as active when gathered too early or too late, as it is when taken at the middle of the flowering season; and whatever circumstances interfere with the usual course of this process, these will alter the quality of the pollen produced.

Whatever may be the nature of the influences which modify the activity or power of pollen in producing hay-fever, this power was always present in a greater or lesser degree in all the plants experimented with. In some it was so mild that it was necessary to repeat the experiment several times and under varying circumstances in order to be certain that it was present. In others the action was both rapid and vigorous, and such that, if continued, would have led to severe suffering, if not to dangerous symptoms.

§ 143. Before proceeding to inquire what particular portion of the pollen grain or what particular substance contained in this is the active agent in producing hay-fever, it will perhaps be well to notice some conditions which seem to have no influence whatever either in bringing on the attacks or in modifying their intensity when once produced.

The pollen grains of different orders of plants vary much in size and in weight; in some cases not being more than one twentieth the size or weight of others. This circumstance, however, does not directly affect their power of producing hay-fever. The size of the pollen grain has no relation to the intensity of the symptoms.* A large pollen grain may produce a mild attack, whilst a smaller one may produce much more severe derangement.

Pollen grains also vary in shape and in the roughness or smoothness of their outer coat. In the state in which the pollen comes to be when in contact with the mucous membrane of the nares, or of the trachea and bronchial tubes, in some cases the outer coat will be perfectly smooth and even,† such as for instance in the cereals or the grasses. In others the surface is studded over with sharp points, as in the order Compositæ; and whatever may be the varying conditions such pollen is placed under, with regard to excess or deficiency of moisture, this roughness is never entirely got rid of. Between these two extreme characters of surface there are all degrees, but in no case have I noticed that the shape, or the degree of roughness of the surface, has any influence in regulating the intensity of the symptoms produced.

We have seen that in the list given there are several plants of a poisonous character. This circumstance, however, seems not to affect the quality of the pollen, so far at any rate as the production of hay-fever is concerned. In one of the most poisonous families (Solaneæ), the pollen produced even milder symptoms than that of the grasses.

§ 144. In commencing the inquiry into the question as to what constituent of pollen is the exciting cause of hay-fever, we encounter some difficulties which are not easily removed. Whatever part the pollen-cell may take in the generation of the varied and beautiful forms of plant life, even with the aid of the most powerful instruments it gives to the vegetable physiologist no indication of the possession of those wonderful powers which belong to it and which lie hidden in its apparently structureless granular matter.

In like manner, if we seek for any sign of pollen being the cause of this disease, we find no special character in

* When equal quantities by weight are applied.
† So far as a magnifying power of 450 diameters will show.

any portion of the cell which will enable us to account for the phenomena of hay-fever.

Pollen is, in its recent state, a living structure, and if we attempt to examine it by chemical means or by any mode of manipulation which alters the relation of its separate parts, we may change its character and lessen its vitality. It will no longer be the active and living organism it was before our examination began, and the changes we have brought about may involve the alteration or destruction of those very qualities upon which the production of morbid phenomena depends. These may and probably do to some extent depend upon the vitality which it possesses in common with all bodies of the same class; consequently in all our examinations we are constantly met by the difficulty there is in keeping intact the disease-producing quality whilst we isolate that portion of the pollen to which it belongs.

There are, however, some of the symptoms of hay-fever which are probably due to mechanical causes, but which are nevertheless produced by pollen.

§ 145. Examined under the microscope a pollen cell is a simple cell with granular contents. Its cell wall is generally composed of two layers only—an *intine* or inner coat and an *extine* or outer coat.* In addition to these two membranes pollen of almost all kinds is covered with a substance which resembles an oleo-resin, and in some instances I have thought that a portion of this substance has come from the interior of the pollen grain. In some cases this oleo-resin is of a rich amber colour, when seen under the microscope, whilst in others it is of a pale straw colour. It varies in quantity in different pollens. In that of *Lilium album* it is especially abundant and also in that of the *Calendula officinalis*, as well as in several other plants of the order Compositæ. It is very little soluble in water or in proof

* There is also a third coat in some pollens. In the pollen of the *Cucurbita ovifera* I have found this third coat to consist of an exceedingly delicate membrane which seems to lie between the inner and outer coat. It is not seen until the pollen has been immersed in water, or in water and glycerine, for two or three days; it then protrudes and lifts up the minute lids which cover the pores in this pollen grain.

spirit, but dissolves readily in ether and in oil of turpentine. I believe it slowly volatilises at ordinary temperatures, but of this I cannot speak very positively. It is this substance which causes pollen to adhere to any body with which it comes in contact when fresh.* Some of the pollens which have the largest quantity of this oleo-resin about them are not so active in producing hay-fever as those which contain much less of it. All the pollens of the grasses that I have examined have a very small quantity about them, and yet they are amongst the most active in producing the symptoms of hay-fever. From these considerations I conclude that this body has little or no influence on the disease, and that we must look to some other portion of the pollen grain for the exciting cause of the malady.

§ 146. Seen under the microscope, when fresh, pollen grains have generally a definite and regular shape. When dried they usually also shrink into a shape more or less regular in character, but in a certain portion of the contents of any anther the dried grain will have the appearance of an amorphous particle of silica. The outer coat is seen to be pierced with small round holes or slits—pores. The inner membrane stretches across these openings and never in any case, so far as I have observed, allows the interior of the cell or its contents to be exposed to the atmosphere until this membrane has been ruptured.

§ 147. When water† is allowed to come into contact

---

* Referring to this subject Lindley says:—" In all cases where there are asperities of the surface or angles in the outline, pollen is asserted by Guillemin to have a mucous surface, which was first observed in Proteaceæ by Brown; but Mohl finds that the presence of mucosity upon pollen is a constant character, at least, when the grains first quit the anther; and that a power of secreting a viscid substance is one of their functions when perfectly smooth, as well as when covered with points and inequalities. He, however, admits that hispid pollen is generally more viscid than that which is smooth." This supposed *mucus*, or *mucosity*, is really the substance, which I have described above. When properly tested, however, it may be found to be a wax and not an oleo-resin, and may possibly be one source from which bees obtain wax for cell-building. Any substance of the nature of mucus would not be soluble in oil of turpentine.—C. H. B.

† Other fluids will also act in a similar manner, but none more quickly than water.

with the dried pollen this quickly swells and assumes its normal shape, and if the quantity of moisture is not too great it will retain its natural shape for a considerable time. If moisture continues to be supplied it loses its form, and whatever may have been its shape previously it tends to become more or less spherical. Carried still further, the granular contents of the cells are seen to alter their position; the inner membrane is seen to protrude more or less through the pores, and to form in this way minute mastoid processes, in some cases bulging very considerably beyond the outer coat. The granular contents will, in the case of the pollens of the grasses, move to the end at which the single pore is, in this pollen, situated, leaving one third or one half of the cell comparatively empty. After a short time, varying according to the condition of the pollen, when placed in contact with water the portion of the granular contents of the cell which is nearest to the pore is expelled with great force—so much so that I have frequently seen a pollen grain driven by degrees half way across the field of the microscope by this expulsive force.*

After the granular matter has escaped it diffuses itself gradually in the surrounding fluid. When carefully observed the granules are seen to vary very much in size. According to Lindley they are, in some cases, not more than the 30,000th of an inch in diameter.† Immersed in

* Lindley says this enlargement and bursting of the pollen grain is the effect of *endosmosis*. This, however, would not force the granular matter to one end of the pollen sac unless some special apparatus, adapted for this purpose, was within the sac. This I believe to be the case. I have on three occasions seen what appeared to me to be a small membranous sac within the inner coat of the pollen grain, and situated at the end farthest from the pore. When the water has been applied for some time, this sac has been seen to expand gradually, and by this expansion to force the granular matter against the end where the pore is situated. After the inner membrane is ruptured and the granular matter has begun to escape the sac seems to collapse or in some way to become so indistinct as not to be seen. I have seen it twice in the pollen of grass and once in that of geranium; but although I have carefully watched for the phenomenon on several other occasions, I have not been able to detect it except in the three instances named. When it is seen it is perceptible for a very short time only.

† Lindley's 'Introduction to Botany,' p. 190.

water or in any fluid which is not of greater density than water they readily take on molecular motion.* This is most perceptible in the smallest granules and seems to be more sluggish as the granules get larger, until in some pollens we find the largest granules to have little or none of this movement. It is said to be caused by the particles "moving on their axes," and setting up in this way a sort of rotary motion. A little observation will, however, show that in addition to this they have a vibratory motion, and that they slowly move in different directions, and sometimes I have noticed that they seem to work together in small groups as if attracted by some force which operates to bring certain of the granules together.†

§ 148. With a solution of *Iodine* the granular matter becomes dark blue, showing by this change that it is an *amyloid* substance. The finer particles colour, in proportion to their size, more deeply than the larger particles. Immersion in antiseptics has no influence on the motion unless these are strong enough to destroy the form of the granules.

Boiling the granular matter, also, does not interfere with the motion, but any liquid more viscid than water lessens the extent of the motion in proportion to the density or viscosity of the liquid. Immersion in glycerine will almost entirely put a stop to it.

§ 149. If instead of bringing the pollen grain into direct contact with water we allow the *vapour* of water to act upon it, the changes described above occur much more

* This was first noticed by Gleichen, and subsequently by Amici, Guillemin, and Brown.

† Molecular motion is seen in almost all animal or vegetable fluids if these are not too viscid to permit the molecules to move. Granular matter is especially abundant and active in vaccine lymph if taken on or before the eighth day, and also in the fluid thrown off by perspiration in rheumatic, typhoid, and other fevers. It is also seen, but to a less extent, in the perspiration of health.

Any watery fluid which holds in suspension finely divided mineral or earthy matter will also show the molecular movement, but in this case I have never found it to be as vigorous or as long continued as it is when the granular matter has been derived from animal or vegetable bodies.

slowly. We reproduce, in fact, the condition in which pollen is placed when it is brought into contact with the respiratory mucous membrane by being inhaled, and we are, with suitable appliances,* able to watch changes such as occur when pollen is brought into contact with the mucous membranes. In the one case, however, we have *mucus* and *watery vapour* acting upon the pollen, whilst in the other we have only watery vapour present. Nevertheless, from what I have been able to learn, by immersing pollen in liquids of similar density and viscosity to those of mucus it is very improbable that the latter has any effect which would not be produced by the vapour given off from the lungs during expiration.

§ 150. The pollen which is found floating in the atmosphere during the prevalence of hay-fever is, as I shall have to show further on, dry and shrivelled. A few minutes' exposure to the air and the sun on a summer's day is sufficient to deprive it of the moisture which it contains in its normal state whilst enclosed within the walls of the anther. If we imitate this action by allowing the pollen to dry before we subject it to the influence of the vapour, we can then observe all the physical changes which take place when pollen is inhaled during the hay season.

---

* One of the readiest methods of observing the changes which occur in pollen under the influence of watery vapour is to use what may, for convevience, be called a *water cell*. This may be constructed in the following manner. A drop of distilled water is placed, whilst still warm, in a microscopic cell about one tenth of an inch deep by half an inch in diameter. The upper surface of the cell wall is coated with black varnish, and this is allowed partially to dry. A disc of thin microscopic glass, on which a portion of fresh pollen has been dusted, is then placed on the cell in the form of a lid, care being taken that the surface on which the pollen has been placed is turned downwards. If the varnish has not been allowed to become too dry the edges of the thin glass will adhere to it, and thus a cell will be formed which is hermetically sealed. Care should also be taken that the water is only just sufficient to cover the bottom of the cell.

If it is desired to have the pollen as a permanent preparation after the changes have taken place in it, it is necessary to leave two or three spaces on the surface of the cell wall untouched with varnish. The water will then slowly evaporate, and the changed condition of the pollen is rendered permanent.

As I have said above, one of the first changes is that the pollen grain begins to swell. In contact with water this is accomplished somewhat suddenly, but under the influence of vapour it is produced more slowly and with accompaniments which may possibly help us to account for some of the phenomena of hay-fever.

The enlargement is not brought about by a steady increase in size. The change is produced in many of the pollen grains by a series of jerks, as if the cell wall resisted for a time the expansive force of the moisture which had condensed around it and then suddenly gave way, and in doing so not only altered its shape but also slightly changed its position. After this change has taken place the granular matter begins to escape, but it does so much more slowly and less vigorously than when in contact with water, though occasionally this sudden and spasmodic mode of exit is seen. In both cases the granules have a tendency to diffuse themselves in the surrounding fluid, but with water they do so more completely than with vapour. In both instances a portion of the matter will remain in contact with the grains, grouped together as if held in close contact by the viscid mucus in which they are imbedded whilst in the pollen grain; the least mechanical disturbance, however, will set a large number of them free, and in such case they at once commence the molecular motion.

If placed under a micrometer* whilst the granular matter is being ejected, the pollen grain is seen to move slowly across the field of the microscope, or if this remains stationary the stream of granules is pushed in an irregular or zigzag line away from it. In some cases a dozen or more pollen grains may be seen undergoing this change in a single field, and when we consider that in the space of one square centimètre ($=\frac{10}{25}$ths of an English inch) we have about six hundred fields, some idea may be formed of the extent of mechanical action which goes on in a comparatively small surface of the mucous membrane of the nares, trachea, and bronchial tubes, during the time when grass is in flower.

* The squares on the micrometer enable us to measure the distance travelled, however small and however slow the movement may be.

§ 151. When pollen is immersed in water, if it is quite ripe some of the grains will burst in a few seconds, others will take an hour or two, and some will not discharge their contents however long they are kept moist. Sometimes the granular matter is seen in close contact with the pollen sac from which it has been ejected. In some instances the contents of a grain may be discharged at a single stroke, whilst in others the evacuation may go on more moderately, and in the latter case it sometimes happens that a large group of granules may partially block up the pore, whilst smaller detachments are being discharged by pushing their way past the side of the larger group.

As in the other case the pollen grains are sometimes seen to move across the field of the microscope, or to push the granular matter from them, but this they generally do more suddenly and more vigorously than when under the influence of vapour only. The granular matter diffuses more rapidly in the surrounding fluid, and the number of granules which take on molecular motion is larger, whilst at the same time this is more vigorous; but the chief difference between the two modes of operating consists in the difference in the time taken to accomplish the results.

The two modes of action described above do, in practice, slide so gradually from one to the other, and become so intermingled, that it is very difficult to ascertain the precise point at which the one ends and the other begins.

At the commencement of an attack the first symptoms will, no doubt, be produced by the combined action of the vapour exhaled from the lungs and the mucus secreted by the mucous membrane. If the quantity of pollen which is brought into contact with the mucous membrane be small, or if its vitality is lessened by any circumstance, this mode of action may be kept up some time, but when a discharge of serum begins we shall at once have the more rapid and vigorous action commenced which is seen when pollen is placed in contact with water. Thus it happens that the fluid which is discharged in great profusion in severe attacks of hay-fever is at once a *cause* and an *effect*; and so

PLATE I.

Fig. 1.

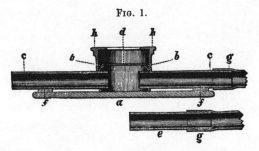

Fig. 1.—A perpendicular section of the instrument represented. *a*, glass plate (one tenth of an inch thick); *b, b*, circular brass cell, cemented to the glass plate *a*, and perforated on opposite sides for the passage of the glass tubes *c, c*, which latter are cemented into the cell *b, b*; *d*, a disc of thin microscopic glass, which rests on the upper margin of the cell *b, b*, the pollen intended for observation being placed on the under surface of this glass; *e*, a short piece of glass tube, to be used as a mouth-piece; *f, f*, brass steps cemented to the upper surface of the glass plate *a*, the tubes *c, c*, being cemented to semicircular recesses in the steps *f, f*; *g*, caoutchouc tube, attached by one extremity to the mouth-piece *e*, and by the other to the tube *c*. This tube should be sufficiently long to reach the mouth of the operator easily when the cell is in position on the stage of the microscope. *h, h*, brass cap to fit over the cell *b, b*. The cap is raised a little, so as to show the disc of thin glass *d*; but when in position, the under surface of the horizontal portion of the cap will press upon the disc and keep it firmly fixed.

Fig. 2.

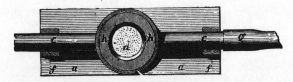

Fig. 2.—A view of the upper surface of Fig. 1. *a, a*, glass plate (an ordinary microscopic slide will answer the purpose); *c, c*, glass or brass tubes cemented to the steps *f, f*, and to the cell *b, b*, which is here concealed by the cap *h, h*; *g*, caoutchouc tube attached to the mouth-piece *e* (shown in Fig. 1), and to the tube *c*; *h, h*, brass cap which holds the disc of glass *d* in position, and covers the cell *b, b* (shown in Fig. 1).

Drawn to a scale of ⅔rds.

long as a free supply of pollen is kept up this fluid helps in
no small degree to perpetuate and to intensify the symptoms
generated.

§ 152. The form of cell which I now use for demonstrating the effect of vapour upon pollen is shown at Figs. 1 and 2. (Plate I.)

A cell of this form possesses several advantages over the simpler one described in the footnote to § 149. One advantage is that the observer can, whilst witnessing the changes which take place under the microscope, accelerate or retard these at pleasure, and can also bring them to a termination at any particular stage. With these exceptions the process followed, in using this instrument, is a pretty close imitation of what takes place when pollen is inhaled.

§ 153. When fresh pollen has been placed on the under surface of the glass disc d, if we breathe gently through the mouthpiece e, the vapour exhaled from the lungs will pass through the cell b, b, and will condense on and around the pollen. By increasing the speed at which the respired air is made to pass through the cell, we may gain a tolerably accurate notion of the rate at which the changes before-mentioned take place in varying rates of respiration.

By this means we shall be able to ascertain that, whilst active exercise must necessarily increase the quantity of pollen inhaled during the hay season, it also greatly accelerates those changes which produce some of the symptoms of hay-fever.

§ 154. If we are desirous of imitating the natural process of respiration in the operation, we can do so by drawing the air in through the cell, and passing it out by the same way.

The only advantage there is in pursuing this method is, that it enables us to determine with tolerable accuracy the time which elapses before the changes, which I have described, are completed.

§ 155. There is also another change brought about in pollen by the influence of vapour which, although it may not have much share in producing the symptoms to which pollen gives rise, it would not be well to pass by without noticing.

So far as relates to the pollen cell itself, when in its normal position, this change is physiological in character; but so far as it relates to the mucous membrane with which the former is in contact, when inhaled, it is purely mechanical.

When pollen is discharged from the anther a considerable portion of it comes into contact with the stigmata of the plant to which it belongs. In this position the inner membrane* of the pollen sac very soon begins to protrude through one of the pores, and eventually becomes elongated into a fine transparent tube (*pollen tube*), which is filled with the granular matter (*fovilla*) of the pollen grain. In fulfilling its proper function this tube passes into or between the cells and tissue which form the stigma.

§ 156. This development of the pollen-tube may be seen to occur in a very small number of the cells, when placed under the microscope, in the instrument shown in Figs. 1 and 2 (Plate I); and there can be very little doubt that the same change takes place when pollen is brought into contact with the mucous membranes of the respiratory passages. Generally the proportion in which the change does occur is very small, and it is only in certain states of the pollen that it is to be seen at all. What the exact nature of this condition is is not at present known.

Occasionally the tube may be seen to grow rapidly, so that in the course of thirty or forty minutes it may grow to a length which is two or three times the diameter of the pollen cell. Whether the tube simply stretches along the surface of the mucous membrane, or whether it penetrates into the mucous follicle, it is impossible at present to say; nor can we feel at all sure that its presence does assist in producing any of the symptoms of hay-fever. I think it is not improbable, however, that it does in some few instances penetrate the mucous follicle, and thus give rise to irritation, which at least increases that set up in other ways.

* It is possible that the inner membrane (*intine*) does not in all cases form the pollen tube, but that in some it is formed by the delicate membrane (*exintine*) of which I have spoken (§ 145). It is also probable that this middle coat may be present in all pollens, though it cannot always be detected.

§ 157. I have thus shown that pollen possesses the power of producing hay-fever, both in its asthmatic and its catarrhal form; and I have also shown that, with very rare exceptions, this power is common, in some degree, to the pollen of all the plants experimented with. And, although those belonging to the order Graminaceæ have this property in a more marked degree than some, there are plants belonging to other orders which have it to almost, if not quite, an equal extent. How far this property would be found to extend through the plants which form the entire flora of any given district I cannot at present say, but I do not doubt that the exceptions would be comparatively few.

From the results obtained in the experiments I have described, I have come to the conclusion that the disturbance caused by pollen is due partly to its mechanical and partly to its physiological action. From the circumstance, however, that the coating of wax or oleo-resin, of which I have spoken (§ 145), probably has some volatile oil combined with it, it is possible that this may commence the disturbance; but whether this is chemical or physiological in its character is not certain.

§ 158. The mechanical changes I have described would be quite sufficient to account for some of the earlier symptoms of hay-fever; but some of the later phenomena will, no doubt, be due to the physiological action of the granular matter of the pollen.

This granular matter, as I have shown at § 147, will, with suitable conditions, take on the Brownian or molecular movement. It might, at first sight, appear likely that this movement would assist in bringing on or in prolonging the symptoms produced by the other mechanical changes. But when we remember that all very small particles or mineral and organic matter will, under similar conditions, take on the same movements,* though not in all cases to

---

* In speaking of the nature and causes of this movement, Valentin says:—
"There can be no doubt that direct mechanical agitation, and indirect thermic movements, exert an important influence on the phenomena we are now considering. And although the results differ with the nature of the molecules and the fluid, still the mutual physical relations may assist to determine the amount

the same extent, we are compelled to think that this can have no share in producing hay-fever. If molecular motion was an efficient cause for any of the important symptoms of the disorder, patients who are liable to it would suffer more or less from it at all times, because experiment has shown that there is an abundance of finely divided matter present in the atmosphere at various parts of the year, independent of any particular season.

§ 159. The power which the granular matter of pollen has may, however, be due to qualities which are very different in their nature. It may, as I have before intimated, depend upon the possession of that vitality which all bodies of this class have in their active state; and the moment this vitality is destroyed the granular matter may, so far as hay-fever is concerned, be rendered quite innocuous. On the other hand, it may, when all the chemical constituents of pollen come to be known, be found, in part at least, to depend upon the presence of a substance belonging to the alkaloid or to some other class of bodies. Until pollen has been subjected to a more careful chemical investigation than it has yet undergone, this part of the question must be considered unsettled. This much, however, may be considered to be tolerably certain, namely, that the sneezing—and possibly the discharge of serum—which occurs in the first stage of hay-fever is due to the mechanical changes of which I have spoken, and that the swelling caused by the effusion of fluid into the submucous cellular tissue is due to the presence of some substance or quality in the granular matter, the exact nature of which is at present unknown.

§ 160. I have found by experiment that the granular matter of pollen may, by dialysis, be made to pass through membranes which are thicker than those which line the air-vesicles and bronchial tubes; and from this circumstance I think that it is highly probable that the finer particles of

of original displacement and the duration of the subsequent vibration. The question whether these are the sole exciting causes, or whether the molecular movement is not based upon other attractive forces cannot at present be decided. The forces to which it is due are, at any rate, easily overcome by the ordinary phenomena of adhesion."—(Vide *Text Book of Physiology*, p. 356.)

this matter do, in some cases, pass through the mucous membrane of the respiratory passages, and by getting into the circulation in this way give rise to the constitutional symptoms we see developed in some cases.* Why it should not be so in all cases is, however, not very clear. In some instances it may be due to the greater power of resistance which some patients have; and in others it may depend upon the quantity and kind of pollen inhaled.

§ 161. There is another supposed cause of a form of hay-asthma to which I have not as yet adverted, namely, the odour given off by certain animals. It is said that the presence of cats, rabbits, or guinea pigs, will in some cases cause a form of asthma which cannot be distinguished from hay-asthma. Although I cannot deny the apparent truth of the statements of those authors who have cited these curious examples of the disorder, I must say that I think it is possible that many of those cases would be found on very close investigation to be capable of being explained in a different way.

I have shown that, when pollen is subjected to the influence of moisture, the pollen sac when ripe bursts and discharges its granular contents. If, in the process of making, the hay has been wet by any means, much of the pollen which is in contact with the partially dried herb will undergo this change, and thus it will happen that, when the hay is completely dried, it will have mixed up with it not only a large number of perfectly formed pollen grains, but also a quantity of the finely divided granular matter in a dried state.

* The granular matter of pollen consists, in part, of what Beale would call *vegetable bioplasm.* The smallest particles probably consist almost entirely of this material, but the larger particles have a portion of *formed material* combined with it.

Beale is entirely opposed to the idea that any bioplasm of vegetable origin can be the cause of contagious disease.[1] In the present state of our knowledge it is unwise to dogmatise too persistently on this question. I have shown that one form of vegetable matter can give rise to a disease which is not transmissible, and it is not impossible that a vegetable bioplasm may yet be found which can play the part of a $\zeta\acute{v}\mu\eta$ after it has obtained an entrance into the circulation, and thus set up some form of contagious disease.

---

[1] Vide *Disease Germs: their supposed Nature,* p. 9.

§ 162. Now, in the case of the two last named animals, it is well known that they are often kept almost constantly amongst hay, and in the case of the first its excursions in search of mice are often made in lofts where large quantities of hay are stored, and it may therefore with very great propriety be suggested that the fur of these animals may be simply the carrier of the granular matter and of the pollen.

Although I have made most diligent inquiry, I have never yet met with a case in which the attacks could be shown to be due entirely to the odour given off by animals; but, nevertheless, I am not prepared to say that no such cases exist, and only desire to offer the facts named above as a possible explanation of some of the attacks which are said to be caused by animal odours.

G. *Observations on the influence of light and heat.*

§ 163. Light has been referred to by Dr. Phœbus and other writers on hay-fever as one of the probable causes of the disorder; but on what ground this assertion has been made does not appear. Light is one of the most universally diffused agents we have. We have abundant evidence to show the important influence it has in aiding those changes which make up the sum total of life in the animal and vegetable kingdom, but we have no evidence to show that it has the power to produce symptoms which have even a remote resemblance to those of hay-fever, and, so far as I am aware, no author has yet made experiments which prove that light can produce the fully developed disease.

Both light and heat have been thought by some authors, and also by some patients, to give rise to exacerbations of the disorder, when once it has been established, but we have no evidence to show that the actual exciting cause of the disease has not been present when these exacerbations have come on, apparently through exposure to light. Then, again, it has not been proved that the period at which we have the greatest average intensity of light is the period at which hay-fever prevails. Until evidence, which will clear up these uncertainties, is brought we shall be justified in refusing to accept the statements of those who maintain that light is one of the causes of hay-fever.

§ 164. The powerful influence which heat has in deranging the whole economy of the animal frame has been recognised from very early times, but in searching the works of writers on medicine, and especially of those who have treated upon the action of heat as a cause of disease, we look in vain for any description of symptoms resembling those of hay-fever. The derangements produced by exposure to intense heat are, in fact, very different in character and severity to those we observe in catarrhus æstivus. But notwithstanding this, the ill-recognised changes which heat produces on the nervous and vascular systems seem to have attracted the attention of some authors who were wishful to find a powerful cause for this curious disorder. Other authors have followed in the wake of these, and in some cases have adopted their conclusions without ascertaining the nature of the evidence upon which these rest.

§ 165. Bostock was, as we have seen (§ 33), the first to ascribe the malady to the influence of heat. His experiments seem at first sight to bear out his conclusions, but when we closely examine the evidence he brings we find that the former were not very logical.

The principal thing that strikes us in these observations is the circumstance that although heat was thought by Bostock to be the sole cause of his disorder, he passed through two of the hottest summers (1825-26) we have had during the present century and had fewer attacks of the disease than was usual in ordinary years. Again, in the first year of his residence at Ramsgate (1824) the summer was not warmer than usual, and yet he does not say that he suffered less than in the two hot summers.

§ 166. If his theory was correct and he had the disorder in so mild a form during the hot weather, he ought to have been almost entirely free from it in the cooler weather of 1824. If this had been the case one would think he would not have failed to notice the fact, since he tells us he made choice of Ramsgate as a residence in order to try to lessen the severity of the attacks. He, however, does not say he escaped or that he had the disease in a milder form even, and we are, therefore, led to infer that he must have suffered in the usual way during the first summer.

It is true that Bostock believed that the cooler air of the sea coast was the cause of the comparative immunity he enjoyed during the two hot summers. There is, however, not a sufficient difference between the temperature of the air in this situation and at a distance from the sea, to account for the non-occurrence of the attacks at the former place. Bostock says that whenever he walked out, or, as he terms it, "relaxed his plan of discipline" he was sure to have an attack. But the average temperature of the air in a room would, during such summers as we had in 1825 and 1826, be quite equal to what it is in ordinary years in the open air, and it is well known that hay-fever is quite as severe at such times as it is in very hot summers. It has, in fact, sometimes happened that I have had the disorder in a milder form in a hot and very dry summer than I have when the air has been cooler and more moist. The year 1868 was, so far as the neighbourhood of Manchester is concerned, a fair example of the kind of summer which tends rather to lessen than to increase the severity of hay-fever.

§ 167. The year 1827 was cool, and during this summer Bostock resided at Kew, and whilst there he "walked out daily in the midst of hundreds of acres of meadow-grass," yet, except during one or two hot days in July, he had no attacks. This experience seems to favour his theory much more than that gained by his residence at Ramsgate. I have, however, shown (§ 142) that in a cool summer very little pollen is formed by grass, and I shall be able to show as I pass on that a rise in the temperature, during the hay season, will sometimes cause large quantities of pollen to be formed and thrown off.

It has several times in the course of my experiments seemed during a period of comparative coolness of the atmosphere, if the temperature has not gone down too low, as if the pollen has been, as it were, reservoired for a time, and as soon as the temperature has risen beyond a certain point the accumulated stock has been rapidly thrown off. But, however, this may be, certain it is that heat and moisture favour the growth and evolution of pollen and that cold and dryness will almost completely put a stop to these processes.

§ 168. As it bears upon this part of the subject I will mention here an incident which occurred to me at Filey in 1870. This occurrence shows the manner in which attacks of hay-fever may come on even at the sea-side, and it also shows how careful we should be in forming our opinions before we have investigated all the circumstances attending an attack.

It was on one of the hottest days which occurred in July that I went down to the sea-shore for the purpose of trying some of the experiments named at § 97. The day was very hot, a sea breeze was blowing at the time and had been blowing more or less for two days. I was quite free from any of the active symptoms of hay-fever at the time. I remained from ten o'clock in the morning till five in the afternoon, moving about on the cliffs or on the shore close to the water. At the termination of the day's experimentation I returned to the town by a field-path which leads to the older part of the town. I had not proceeded far along this path before some of the earlier symptoms of hay-fever began to show themselves, and in the course of a very short time a violent attack of sneezing and coryza came on. So sudden and, so far as the action of pollen appeared to be concerned, so causeless was the attack that I began to think that after all there might be occasions in which light, heat, ozone, or all combined, might bring on hay-fever. I had only just quitted the sea-shore, and there was only a comparatively narrow strip of cultivated land intervening between me and the sea. On searching, however, I found that on this narrow belt of land there was a field of wheat in full bloom, and, on examining closely, the ripe anthers could be seen to be ejecting their pollen in the way which may frequently be witnessed in many families of plants, and especially in those belonging to the order Graminaceæ.* It is scarcely necessary to say that as soon as I got away from the wheat the symptoms which had shown themselves so suddenly began to abate.

§ 169. I had here a fair opportunity of testing the action of light, heat, ozone and pollen. After several hours' exposure to the three agents first named no effect was produced, but in the case of the pollen I had not been in contact with it many minutes before its characteristic symptoms began to be developed.

In order to be quite sure that the sea air did not carry any pollen, a short series of experiments—six in number— were tried by a method which I shall have to describe in the next chapter. By these experiments I found that when the wind had been blowing in from the sea for some hours, if the instrument was placed closed to the margin, and a few feet above the surface, of the water the air did not contain any pollen or any solid matter whatever. I was therefore satisfied that the absence of the symptoms of hay-fever during the greater part of the day was due to the absence of pollen, and that its sudden occurrence in the latter part of the day was due to a temporary exposure to its influence at the spot named.

§ 170. As I have before intimated when speaking of the experiments on ozone, this particular spot (Filey Bay) was selected because we have here an expanse of ocean which stretches three to four hundred miles in a straight line from the English coast; so that when the wind blows in from the sea a sufficient length of time to insure its having crossed the entire distance, we have here a fair opportunity for determining whether pollen or other organic matter can cross large tracts of ocean.

* If an ear of one of the Graminaceæ with large anthers (Rye, for instance) be placed, whilst in full flower, in a vase of water, or in a portion of wet earth or sand, and left in a room where the air is kept moderately still, some of the anthers may be seen to discharge their pollen in a sort of jet, which is thrown out at short intervals. It seems as if only a portion of the anther opens at once and discharges a part of its contents by the action of some *vis a tergo* which causes the pollen to be thrown a line or two in advance of the spot it would occupy if it dropped perpendicularly. What the cause of this mode of ejection is is not easy to make out.

In this case we have seen that the sea air was free from any form of solid matter; but it is important to observe here that under some circumstances it will not be found to be so. In cases, for instance, where the air passes only a short distance over the sea, we shall often have it charged with solid matter; and where a land breeze is driven back after having crossed the sea a little way only, this may carry back the matter it has brought from the coast. In cases, also, where a land wind is driven back after having crossed the ocean a short distance, and where this return current comes back by a path different from that taken in its outward course, the matter it contains may be thrown upon a part of the coast quite different to that from which it came. Thus we may have the products of one part of a continent distributed to another and totally different part.

We know so very little of the modes in which small particles of matter may be transported by atmospheric currents, or of the distances to which these may travel, that it is unwise to presume that they are absent at any time unless they are proved to be so by careful experiment.

§ 171. Bostock seems not to have had any idea of the existence of facts such as those I have just mentioned, and consequently is not at all influenced by them in drawing his conclusions.

Other writers who have treated of the disease since Bostock's time have, as we have seen (Chap. II), attributed it to the influence of heat. Dr. Phœbus, as I have previously shown, has to resort to the curious hypothesis which makes the *early heats* of summer the most active cause of the malady, and speaks of this idea as being supported by the testimony of numerous and important observers.

If this hypothesis is intended to be used in a *qualitative* sense only, then it should be shown that solar heat does possess a property in the early part of the summer which it loses at the later part; and, although it might be impossible to demonstrate the exact nature of this property, its effects should be capable of being shown by experiments made at a time when no other supposed cause of hay-fever is present. If, however, the hypothesis is intended to be used only in a *quantitative** sense, it should, as I have said before, be shown that an increase of temperature beyond a certain point invariably brings on the disorder. In no case has this yet been done.

§ 172. Dr. Smith agrees with Dr. Phœbus in believing that great heat and strong light will induce or aggravate the symptoms of hay-fever, but he does not bring us the history of any cases which show conclusively that these agents have the power they are said to have. One case, however, is given in which the attack came on whilst the patient was engaged in unfurling the sails of a yacht a short distance out at sea.† In this case it seemed as if heat and physical exertion had brought on the disorder. The experiments I shall have to describe in the next chapter will, however, show that it is highly probable that the sails had become the receptacles for pollen which had been blown on to them from the land, and that the unfurling of the sails had disturbed the pollen and caused it to be inhaled during the period of exertion.

Another case is given by Dr. Smith in which the symptoms of the disorder came on whilst the patient was walking through Piccadilly (London) on a hot, dry, dusty day.‡ The intense heat and the dust, Dr. Smith thinks, were quite sufficient to account for the sudden appearance of the attack. Unless, however, it can be shown that the patient had been suddenly and temporarily brought under the influence of these agents, we shall be warranted in doubting the correctness of this conclusion; and I am myself the more inclined to do so from the circumstance that I have several times had similar sudden attacks when there seemed to be no probability of these being due to pollen, but which were found to be so when a close examination of the attendant circumstances was made. One example of such an occurrence is given at § 118, and another at § 169.

§ 173. Dr. Smith also gives several examples of the

---

* Or merely to indicate intensity.

† *On Hay-fever, or Summer Catarrh*, by W. Abbots Smith, M.D. London, 1866, p. 50.

‡ *Ibid.*, p. 52.

disorder in which the attacks were undoubtedly due to the presence of hay or of grass in flower. For the details of these I must refer my readers to Dr. Smith's work,* but I may be allowed to remark here that the examples of this class of cases are greatly in excess of those that are said to be due to heat.

§ 174. Dr. Pirrie gives a number of cases where the patients attributed their attacks to the heats of summer. One of these patients, in describing the circumstances under which an attack would sometimes come on, says, "Any day I have occasion to be out in summer under a strong sun I am sure to have an attack of the complaint. I am always best in cold, cloudy days in summer."†

Another patient says, "I cannot go out on a very bright hot day without being so ill, and I think it is more from the general effect of heat on me than anything else."‡ Another patient, a lady, told Dr. Pirrie that "she was always ill for many weeks, and was always worst when the season was a bright and sunny one."§ The case of an Indian officer is also mentioned who, while in England, had his attacks at the beginning of June, but who on one occasion was seized when out at sea."‖

Another example of the effect of heat is given where the patient was also an officer in the Indian army. In this case the disease "showed itself in England in the months of June and July. When in India the attacks were more frequent during the whole course of the year than in England, and the worst time for it was from the end of July to the end of September." The patient, however, remarks that "during the hottest season, from March to June, in western India, vegetation is dried up, and the sneezing would be constant enough if excited by the sun."¶

§ 175. From the circumstance that the disease makes its appearance at different times, which accord with the

* *On Hay-fever, or Summer Catarrh,* by W. Abbots Smith, M.D. London, 1868, 4th Edition. Pages 26, 27, 35, 36, and 40.
† *On Hay-asthma and the Affection termed Hay-fever,* by William Pirrie, M.D. London, 1867, p. 28.
‡ *Ibid.,* p. 29. § *Ibid.,* p. 29 ‖ *Ibid.,* p. 30. ¶ *Ibid.,* p. 33.

time at which summer is said to commence in the various districts, Dr. Pirrie thinks " all this has a direct relation to the advent of the hot summer days." He also says, in referring to the occurrence of the disease in India, " it appears in the hot dry weather from March to June ; but also in the period intervening between the end of July and the end of September, but it has also been said to have appeared among Europeans in India during the months of February and March, and then it has been attributed by some to the blossom of mango and some other trees which are then in flower."*

Dr. Moore in his pamphlet agrees with the three last-mentioned authors in attributing the disorder in many cases to the influence of heat, but no cases are given by him in support of this opinion.

§ 176. No author but Dr. Phœbus makes any distinction between the earlier and later heats of summer; and, with all except this writer, it is more a question of intensity than of quality.

When we come, however, to inquire into the effect of heat in countries where the temperature rises far above what we have in England, we find that the experience of the disease gained in these hot countries, gives no countenance to the opinions held by some authors on the effects of heat.

Since the information contained in § 65 was sent to me, the patient whose case is there mentioned has spent several years in the United States. In one of these years she resided at Salem, on the shores of Lake Erie, and here she had the disease just as in England. In speaking of this she says—" I arrived here the first week in May, and, as usual, it was at its worst in June, bad in July, better in August, and well in September."

In the two following years the summers were spent in South Carolina, and here, although the heat must have been much greater than in England, or on Lake Erie, the patient " had not the slightest vestige of an attack." The

* *On Hay-asthma and the Affections termed Hay-fever*, by William Pirrie, M.D. London, 1867, p. 49.

cause of this she believes to be "the small proportion of grass and no hay-making."

Sir Ranald Martin, in speaking of the hot dry season, which, in Bengal, extends from the beginning of March to the middle of June, says, "The temperature rises gradually from 80° to about 90°—95° in the shade, and reaches to 100°—120°—130° in the open air. . . . . . Of Calcutta it may be said, however, with truth that it is 'a city of stone, in a land of iron, with a sky of brass,' the soil of the surrounding country being rent and riven as if baked over a volcano. . . . . . . The local newspapers of May, 1851, speak of the heat as more intense than it has been for years. The thermometer in the coolest rooms stands at 92° to 94°, and the breeze which should bring refreshment at the close of a sultry day has been as the breath of a furnace."*

§ 177. If heat would produce hay-fever, it would, with those who are liable to it, be certain to be developed in India under such circumstances as those described above. But not only should the disease be developed, but it should also be continuous and severe whilst the temperature is high. Such, however, is seldom or never the case. In the few cases which do occur, the intensity of the disorder does not at all correspond with the degree of heat.

A native medical practitioner, educated in England, in answer to inquiries made through a friend, informs me that he has never known a patient—either native or foreign—to be affected with hay-fever in the plains, and he believes that the disease has never been known to occur in natives either on the plains or in the hills.

Two medical friends—surgeons in the Indian Service—also inform me that during a residence of some years in India, they have never known the disease to occur in the plains.

§ 178. Then if we turn to the evidence furnished by patients who have had hay-fever in India, we find that

* *Influence of Tropical Climates in producing the Acute Endemic Diseases of Europeans*, by Sir James Ranald Martin, C.B., F.R.S. London, 1861, pp. 42, 43.

whilst they have mostly escaped it on the plains, they have often had attacks when they have ascended into the cooler atmosphere of the hills (§ 64); and when patients have had it in both situations, although there are some exceptions, the general testimony is that they have had it less severely in the former than they have in the latter place.

The cause of this difference is not very far to seek. During the hot season in India, vegetation is almost burnt up in the plains, whilst in the hills grass and many of the cereals are grown in abundance, and flower and throw off their pollen just as they do in European countries,* and where the disease does occur in the plains it is tolerably certain that it is caused by the pollen of the grasses or of other plants which are in flower at the time.

Patient 4 (§ 67), in answer to my inquiry respecting the time at which he suffered from the disease in India, says:—"It has usually come on after the rains, when the grass is in flower."

The same gentleman, in a letter† written to the editor of the *Lancet*, in describing his case, says:—"My earliest acquaintance goes back to school days, where I was at first suspected of malingering. . . . . From that time, however, up to 1868 (a period of some thirty-five years), when in Kurrachee, I suffered regularly every summer as it came round. Kurrachee during the months of susceptibility, viz., June, July, and August, possesses an unusually constant damp and windy climate from the south-west monsoon. It is situated with the sea in front, and a howling desert around it; not a blade of grass visible; a barren, sandy, and rocky soil, treeless and verdureless, with no green thing,

---

* Dr. Joseph D. Hooker, of Kew, has kindly given me the following information respecting the grasses and cereals which grow in the Himalaya. In answer to my inquiries Dr. Hooker says:—"None of the English grasses which you mention are indigenous to the Himalaya, but some occur there sparingly as escapes. With regard to the native grasses, they are legion; many of them are of the same genus as European, and if hay-fever is due to grasses in England it would be so in Himalaya. Of Himalayan cereals they cultivate wheat and barley, and, more sparingly, oats; also abundantly, maize, rice, millet, &c., as in the south of Europe."

† Dated Kurrachee, February, 1872. Vide *Lancet*, March 23, 1872.

'Where the bird dare not build,
Nor insect wing flit o'er the herbless granite.'

Since my sojourn in it, however, in 1868 (including two years spent in England), I have been quite free from any return of hay-fever."

§ 179. If we look to the symptoms produced by heat in tropical countries, we find these also to differ very materially from those seen in attacks of hay-fever. Sir Ranald Martin, from whose work I have already quoted, gives the following description of the sun-fever—heat apoplexy—of tropical climates:—" First, we have vertigo and headache, with sense of burning in the eyes, the conjunctiva being injected; a full and frequent pulse, vomiting, great heat, sometimes floridness, of the skin, a devouring thirst, oppressed respiration, and swollen face. Then come lividness, sinking and running of the pulse, clammy sweat, exhausted nervous energy, faltering of the tongue, coma, convulsion, and speedy death ; these constitute the course of events in true heat apoplexy."*

In character as well as in severity the symptoms here given will, when we come to consider those of catarrhus æstivus, be found to be very unlike those which are present in this disorder. To this, however, I shall return in another chapter.

§ 180. The experience we have of the disorder in England agrees in the main with that obtained in India. It is well known that the disease often makes its appearance here before the summer has fairly commenced, and in a very large majority of cases it begins to decline, and frequently entirely disappears, at least for a time, whilst the summer heat is nearly at its maximum. A second attack will also sometimes come on in the autumn, when the temperature is considerably lower than it is during the first attack.

In England also patients generally suffer more severely in the country than they do in the towns, but it is no where contended that the heat of a town is very much

---

* *Influence of Tropical Climates in producing the Acute Endemic Diseases of Europeans*, by Sir James Ranald Martin, C.B., F.R.S., p. 397.

less than that of the country in the summer time; and it is well known that some patients remain almost entirely free from the disease if they reside in the centre of a large town or city during the hay season. A sojourn at the sea-side, too, whatever the temperature may be, will in almost all cases free the patient from the disorder whilst a sea breeze is blowing.*

§ 181. A careful search through the works and published papers of all the authors with whose writings I have become acquainted has shown me that in no instance has it ever been satisfactorily demonstrated that the disease was due to heat, and heat only.

It is true that many cases are given where heat seems to have been the exciting cause, but in not one of these has it been shown that the real exciting cause, pollen, has been absent.

The results of the experiments I shall have to detail in the next chapter have shown me that this proof is always needed in order to make the evidence at all conclusive.

From a consideration of all the facts I have named, and from all the testimony I have gained from the writings of the various authors I have consulted, as well as from that furnished by my own observation and experiments, I am led to conclude that heat has no direct influence in producing hay-fever; and, to use the words I have already quoted, I believe "the cause cannot be anything which is present in other cases where the given effect is not produced, unless the presence of some counteracting cause shall appear to account for its non-production."†

---

* Except under the circumstances named at § 171.
† Archbishop Thomson's *Outline of the Laws of Thought*.

CHAPTER IV.

ON THE QUANTITY OF POLLEN FOUND FLOATING IN THE ATMOSPHERE DURING THE PREVALENCE OF HAY-FEVER, AND ON ITS RELATION TO THE INTENSITY OF THE SYMPTOMS.

A. Experiments at ordinary levels.
B. Experiments at high altitudes.

A. *Experiments at ordinary levels.*

§ 182. We have seen in the preceding pages that pollen can produce the symptoms of hay-fever, but no one hitherto has attempted to show what relation there is between the quantity of pollen found in the air during the prevalence of the disorder and the intensity of the symptoms in any given case.

The researches of Needham and Spallanzani during the last century, and of Boussingault, Pouchet, Pasteur, Schrœder, Salisbury, and others* during the present century, have shown that organised vegetable matters are found floating in the atmosphere. Pollen has frequently been found amongst these matters, but no one has thought it worth while to see what quantity was to be found in any given volume of air or during any given portion of time. Nor yet has any one attempted to determine what family of plants furnishes the largest number. The greatest uncertainty has prevailed on this subject, and this, no doubt, has led to many of the contradictory statements which have

* Crookes, Samuelson, Tyndall, Angus Smith, Dancer, Maddox, Charlton Bastian, &c.

been made on the influence of heat, but which would not have been made if our knowledge of atmospheric deposits had been as complete as it ought to have been.

§ 183. It seemed highly probable that grass pollen would be largely in excess of all others, and that this would be the principal cause of a disorder which prevails mostly during the hay season; but without carefully conducted experiments no correct estimate could be made of the quantity of this pollen to be found in the atmosphere nor yet of the share which other pollens might have in developing the disorder.

Dr. Phœbus in referring to this part of the subject, says, "It is a question whether we have to seek the exciting cause of the whole attack in those atmospheric conditions or in those matters which are found floating in the atmosphere, which we shall speak of as decided causes of aggravation. It is, however, scarcely probable that they, passing more or less quickly, contribute considerably to the creation of the attack—an attack which recurs periodically for life. The scantiness of the causes would, we should think, stand in a disproportion to the greatness of the effect."

Like Dr. Phœbus, I was at first disposed to think that the quantity of pollen in the atmosphere was too small and too quickly passing to produce the effects we see developed in hay-fever. One or two imperfect trials convinced me, however, that this idea was not correct, and I therefore determined to put the matter to the test of a careful investigation.

§ 184. The object of the experiments then was:—

1st. To determine whether the commencement of the disorder depended on the presence of pollen in the atmosphere.

2nd. To ascertain what number of pollen grains would be deposited on a given space each day during the prevalence of hay-fever.

3rd. To determine the height to which pollen would rise and the distance to which it might be transported by atmospheric currents.

4th. To discover what relation the quantity of grass pollen bears to that furnished by other orders of plants.

5th. To see what relation the quantity of pollen found had to the severity of the symptoms produced.

§ 185. The first experiments were made with a very simple apparatus. A glass tube twelve inches long and three quarters of an inch in diameter was filled with air taken in the open country during the hay season, and after having a disc of thin microscopic glass placed at one end so as to stop up the lower orifice, the tube was placed in a perpendicular position, and was allowed to remain quiescent a sufficient length of time to permit any solid particles the enclosed air might contain to deposit on the thin glass. In order to be able to judge of the relative number of pollen grains deposited, a cell, one centimètre square, was formed on the disc with black varnish. Subsequently a metal tube four feet long and an inch and a quarter in diameter was used.

My object in proceeding in this manner was to see what was the smallest quantity of air that would give any reliable results, but in neither case did I find these at all satisfactory. Occasionally the microscope revealed the presence of pollen grains on the disc of glass; but frequently, when I found none in this situation, I could find them on the dust which settled on the inner surface of the tube, and I always found a deposit of some kind on both the glass and metal tubes in spite of all the care that was taken to keep them exactly perpendicular. I could only account for this by supposing that the friction of the external air gave rise to an electric condition of the tube which caused the smaller particles of matter to be attracted by it. Whatever was the cause it helped to defeat the object of the experiments. As a test of the presence of pollen this plan failed as often as it succeeded, whilst as a test of quantity it was an utter failure.

§ 186. Another method which I tried was to draw a given quantity of air through an aspirator, and in doing so to cause the stream of air to impinge against a glass plate covered over with a thin layer of glycerine. The current of air was made to pass through a small tube fixed with the nozzle almost close to the glass plate.*

* Similar to the arrangement adopted by Dr. Maddox in the apparatus invented by him. In his instrument, however, there is no aspirator used. The air is made to pass through the tube by the force of the wind.

Another method which was tried was that which had previously been used by M. Pasteur in his researches on spontaneous generation. The aspirator was made to draw the air through a tube in which was placed a portion of gun cotton; this latter acting as a filter by retaining the particles of solid matter in its meshes. By dissolving the gun cotton in ether, and allowing the particles to settle, these could be seen under the microscope.

Another plan was to fix a piece of thin fine muslin over one end of a tube attached to the aspirator. This muslin was previously moistened with glycerine, but to such a degree that the threads only would be saturated, whilst the square openings between the threads were left patent. When the aspirator was set to work the air was drawn through the muslin, and whatever solid particles this had in it, if they were not small enough to pass through the meshes, they were at once arrested.

§ 187. All these methods answered well as tests of the presence of solid bodies in the atmosphere, but as tests of the quantity they were too difficult, and occupied too much time in the working to permit me to adopt them. In the first plan there was a difficulty in determining whether the whole of the pollen in the air drawn through the tube adhered to the plate charged with glycerine. Unless this could be determined with certainty the plan was really useless as an indicator of quantity. In the second method the trouble involved and the time taken made it impossible to work it, with the time I had at my disposal.

Another plan which was adopted was to aspirate the air through a given quantity of fluid, and then to examine a portion of this under the microscope. A single drop was found to be sufficient to make three or four cells, each of one centimétre square,* and although this method promised at first to be the most scientific and reliable in its results, it was found to be more uncertain and more tedious than any of the other methods.

* The smallest quantity of fluid that could be used to aspirate through would make quite one hundred slides, each having about seven hundred microscopic "fields" in it. I found that unless a very large number of slides were counted no dependence could be placed on the result.

PLATE II.

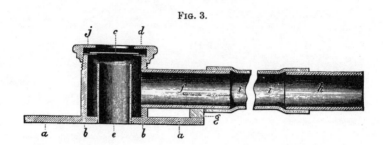

Fig. 3.

Fig. 3.—A perpendicular section of the instrument represented. a, a, brass plate to which the brass cylinder b, b is soldered; c, a square of thin microscopic glass, on which a cell one centimètre square is made with black varnish; d, a loose cap, which screws on to the cylinder b, b. When screwed down, the under and inner surface of this cap rests on small pins, which surround the square of thin glass. e, a smaller cylinder, which is made to screw into the plate a, a; f, a brass or glass tube cemented or screwed into the cylinder b, b; g, brass step screwed to the plate a, a, the tube f being cemented into a semicircular recess on the upper surface of g; h, a short length of glass tube to be used as a mouth-piece; i, i, caoutchouc tube, attached by one extremity to the tube f, and by the other to the mouth-piece h. This tube should be sufficiently long to reach the mouth of the operator when the instrument is placed in position on the stage of the microscope, and the eye of the operator is in position at the eye-piece. A slip of thin glass is shown to be inserted in the tube f; j, a disc of thin brass, perforated with a square opening rather larger than the cell on the thin glass. This disc is made to rest upon the upper edge of the cylinder b, b.

Drawn to a scale of ⅔rds.

PLATE III.

Fig. 4.   Fig. 5.

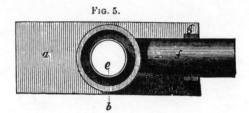

Fig. 4.—A view of the upper surface of the disc of thin brass j. The square of thin glass c is also shown in position.

Fig. 5.—A view of the upper surface of Fig. 3 (the cap d and the disc j being removed). a, brass plate to which the cylinder b is soldered, and into which the smaller cylinder e is screwed; f, glass or brass tube cemented into the cylinder b, and to the step g, g.

When in position the disc j rests on the upper edge of the cylinder b, as shown in Fig. 3. The thin glass c is kept in position by the short pins along its edge, these being screwed into the disc j. The india rubber tube i, i, and the mouth-piece h, are supposed to be removed.

As there is considerable interest taken in the subject of atmospheric deposits at the present time, I have ventured to give a sketch of the various plans adopted, notwithstanding that these were, for the purposes I had in view, almost useless. The record of my failures may, however, possibly prevent other observers, who may think of repeating my experiments, from wasting time in attempting to work in the same way.

§ 188. By an apparatus similar to that shown at Figs. 3, 4, and 5 (Plates II and III), I could ascertain the presence of pollen in the atmosphere at any time, and could form some idea of the quantity inhaled; but the use of this instrument also revealed to me the existence of some disturbing influences and causes of uncertainty, which made it impossible to depend upon experiments tried for short periods.

This instrument I devised for the purpose of viewing the deposit whilst it was forming. By placing it on the stage of the microscope, and inhaling through the mouth-piece h, the glass plate c is for the time being made to take the place of a portion of the mucous membrane of the nares, and the observer can see the deposit as it forms on the field of the microscope. The air being made to enter at the point e, passes up the cylinder and strikes against the thin glass c, this latter being charged with a small portion of the prepared fluid named at § 192. The air then passes over the top of the cylinder e into the tube f, along the tubes ii and h, and into the mouth of the operator.

A slip of thin glass is shown to be inserted in the tube f. This is done with a view of ascertaining what amount of matter escapes being deposited on the plate c. If it is thought to be desirable the caoutchouc tube ii may be divided at different points, and a short length of tube, with a slip of thin glass placed in it, may be inserted. In this way some idea may be formed of the distance to which atmospheric deposits can penetrate into the bronchial tubes. In this case, however, it will be necessary to coat the inner surfaces of the instrument and the tubes with a thin layer of the prepared fluid (§ 192) so as to imitate the condition of the mucous membrane of the buccal cavity, trachea, and bronchial tubes.

§ 189. For observations where it was not deemed necessary to watch the deposit as it formed, a much more simple instrument, constructed on the same principle, was used.*

Either of these instruments seemed at first to be likely to be all that could be desired, but, as in many other cases, the apparent advantages were not found to be so great in practice as they promised. I found that the quantity of pollen in the atmosphere during the hay season was an ever-changing quantity. In no case could I make the product of one, two, or three hours' experimentation agree with the hourly average obtained when the experiments were continued for twenty-four hours at a time. The amount of deposit obtained in a short period was always, or nearly always, largely in excess of the average for a longer period. The deposit obtained in the day was generally much in excess of that obtained during the night. Occasionally, however, the night deposit would be large, whilst that of the following day would be small in amount.

If it had been possible for me to have attached an aspirator to the instrument, and to have kept this constantly going,

---

* This consists of a glass tube six or eight inches long, and rather less than an inch in its inside diameter. This tube is fitted with a square cork sufficiently large to permit it to slide easily into the tube when a moderate force is applied, and yet to remain fixed at any point when untouched. To one end of the tube a brass cap is fitted. This is furnished with an opening rather less than one square centimetre in size. On one surface of the cork a slip of thin glass is fastened by means of two small staples made with thin wire, and placed so as to secure two opposite corners of the glass. If the experiment is intended to be made for the purpose of determining the exact amount of pollen or other deposit a certain number of inspirations will give, it will be necessary to form a cell upon the thin glass in the manner shown at Fig. 6.

When all are in position the cork, with its thin glass, should be about a quarter of an inch from the opening in the brass cap; and this latter should be made to correspond exactly with the position of the cell on the glass.

If air is drawn through the instrument by placing the free extremity of the tube in the mouth of the operator, much the same result may be obtained as with the instrument shown at Fig. 3, with this exception, that the deposit cannot be viewed whilst forming. The slip of glass can be taken out for examination, and should be placed on an ordinary glass slide, so that the lines forming the boundaries of the cell will be parallel to those described by working the screws of the microscope stage. The mode of examining a deposit obtained in this and other ways I shall give further on.

some of these difficulties might have been obviated; but as one series of the experiments had to be conducted in the country, some three miles away from my own residence, this was not practicable.

§ 190. Then there were other difficulties and irregularities which even this would not have obviated. I found, for instance, that a very slight alteration in the position of the instrument, or in the position of the observer, would make a considerable difference in the amount of the deposit, and, as a matter of course, an equal difference in the quantity inhaled. The shelter of a hedge or wall would lessen the quantity perceptibly if the instrument or the patient were placed to the leeward; whilst a wood or large plantation would diminish it more than one half if the trees were in full leaf.

Then, again, I found that the force of the wind made some difference in the amount of pollen deposited. A quiet state of the atmosphere in the height of the hay season generally gave a large amount, but a strong wind lessened the quantity. In the latter case, however, if the wind was not *very* strong, I found the ophthalmic suffering to be more severe than in a quieter state of the atmosphere.

The centre of the city, as might be expected, gave a very much smaller deposit than was got in the country, and as my duties frequently called me into the city whilst the experiments were going on in the country, this introduced another element of uncertainty.

§ 191. Another and very important cause of irregularity was the occurrence of rain during the hay season. If this was very local, and confined to a comparatively small area in the district where the experiments were going on, it would lessen, or entirely put a stop to, the deposit of pollen in this district; but if my duties called me into a part of the country where there had been little or no rain, I should have the symptoms well developed notwithstanding that not a single pollen grain might be shown with the instrument in my own neighbourhood.

§ 192. Ultimately, I was led to adopt a very simple plan, which I afterwards found was recommended by Dr. Phœbus.*

* And has also been used by Dr. Salisbury and other observers.

This consists in the exposure of slips of glass to the open air for a given length of time, so as to allow any solid matter the air may contain to deposit upon the glass. Each slip of glass had a cell formed upon it with black varnish, so as to enclose a space one centimètre square.* This square was coated with a thin layer of fluid prepared for the purpose.† After being exposed for twenty-four hours, each slip was placed under the microscope, and any deposit it contained was carefully examined, and the number of pollen grains counted.

The apparatus on which the glass slips were exposed is shown at Figs. 6 and 7 (Plate IV).

The ultimate object of these experiments was of course to determine as nearly as possible what number of pollen grains floated in the air during each twenty-four hours of a period fixed upon.

At first sight it would appear that this apparatus was not very well adapted for this purpose, and, if very exact estimates are sought for, the remark would be quite true. I found, however, in practice, that this plan of proceeding gave me much more even and reliable results than I had been able to get by any other method, and although they were not quite as exact as might have been desired, they were such as answered well the purposes I had in view.

193. As it was obviously impossible to remain in one spot and thus avoid some of the irregularities of which I have spoken, I determined to use the form of instrument shown above so as to imitate some of the conditions which I have mentioned as the causes of irregularity in the quantity of pollen to which a patient may be exposed in his daily routine.

By a reference to Figs. 6 and 7 it will be seen that there are four slips of glass exposed. Whichever way the wind happens to be blowing, one of these must be more or less under the shelter of the central pillar *b*, and it was astonishing to see what an amount of difference even this little

---

* As shown at Fig. 4.

† In the following proportions:—One part of water, two of proof spirit, and one part of glycerine. Five grains of pure carbolic acid are dissolved in each ounce of this mixture.

PLATE IV.

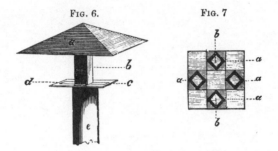

Fig. 6.—*a*, roof or cover to the stage *d*; *b*, pillar which supports the roof *a*; *c*, glass slips seven eighths of an inch square; *e*, socket which fits on to the upper part of a pillar of wood four feet six inches long, and which has its lower extremity fixed into a block of wood which rests on the ground.

Fig. 7.— A view of the upper surface of the stage *d*, the cover *a* being removed; *a, a, a, a,* slips of glass seven eighths of an inch square, on which the cells *b, b* are formed by the borders of black varnish.

Drawn to a scale of ⅕th.

shelter made in the quantity of pollen deposited. During the hay season a patient must, in moving about, be necessarily exposed to similar variations, in some cases amounting to a complete escape from the influence of pollen, and in others to contact with a large quantity. But these variations will often occur under circumstances which will not permit the keenest observer to discover the cause of them.

§ 194. In making these experiments it was not only desirable to pursue a method which would be comparatively easy and which would give results that could be depended upon, but also that this method should allow of the deposit being examined *in situ* before it had undergone any disturbance.

Whilst, on the one hand, I was satisfied that pollen was the most powerful cause of hay-fever, I was, on the other hand, not certain that other organisms might not be found floating in the atmosphere along with pollen, and that some of these might not help to intensify the symptoms set up by it in the first instance.

§ 195. It was therefore important that the organic matter collected should be subjected to as little manipulation as possible, so that if any delicate organisms were by chance found along with pollen these should be uninjured and remain on the glass as they were first deposited. It was principally for this reason that the plan named at § 189 was adopted.

To accomplish the objects aimed at it was, as I have said before, necessary to form some estimate of the comparative number of the pollen grains to be found in the atmosphere during each twenty-four hours of a given period. To show the exact relation there is between the intensity of the disorder and the quantity of pollen in any given case, it would, as I have before intimated, have been needful for the patient experimented upon to remain on the spot where these experiments were conducted during the whole of the time they were going on.

§ 196. The impossibility of pursuing the inquiry in this very precise manner must always render it difficult to make an exact comparison between the quantity of the *materies morbi* and the intensity of the symptoms produced. It will therefore happen that some allowance will have to be made for the difficulty to which I have just alluded, and for the disturbing influences of which I have previously spoken. Nevertheless when we make due allowance for all these difficulties I think it will be seen that the plan adopted has given results as accurate as the nature of the case admits of.

§ 197. Two sets of experiments were tried with the instruments placed at the average breathing level (four feet nine inches from the ground). The spot selected for the first set of experiments was a meadow about fifteen acres in extent, and was situated about four miles to the south-west of Manchester. This land had been used for the growth of hay-grass for more than half a century.

In the first part of the experiments the slips of glass were placed in various situations. In some cases they were sheltered by a hedge or wall, in others by the trunk of a tree or by a gate post. In many cases, however, the glasses were placed in the open field.

§ 198. The quantity of pollen obtained in these different positions was very variable. After a short time the instrument shown at figs. 6 and 7 (Plate IV) began to be used, and although the quantity of pollen was not quite so variable, the number was never the same on all the four glasses. The glass which was placed to the windward of the central pillar invariably contained a much larger number of pollen grains than the one which was placed to the leeward, except where the wind had gone round from one side to the other whilst the experiment was going on; curiously enough, however, the glasses placed in the other two positions rarely contained the same amount of pollen. Probably this arose also from some variation in the direction of the wind.

§ 199. At first the glasses were dry when exposed, but I soon found that this plan was a very uncertain one. Occasionally one of the glasses would have little or no pollen upon it, whilst the others would have a fair quantity upon them; and whilst at the same time I myself had suffered from hay-fever to a degree which quite corresponded with the largest quantity of pollen found: the cause of this irregularity I was some time in discovering. I believe now that the pollen was occasionally consumed by insects, as it was not an uncommon occurrence for me to find the scales of some of the Lepidoptera on the slide. In some attempts also which I made to ascertain the exact weight of pollen contained in one anther, the experiment was often spoiled in consequence of the pollen being consumed by the common blowfly.

Then again I found that in the open air a high wind would clear away a considerable portion of the pollen from the dry glass after it had been deposited. To obviate these difficulties I coated the surface of the glass with a mixture of glycerine and water, but this also I found was liable to the depredations of insects, and ultimately I was led to use the fluid the formula for which is given at § 192.*

After I adopted the plan of coating the surface of the cells with this fluid I found it prevented the deposits being disturbed by insects, and I also found the quantity of pollen to be rather less variable. The glasses were exposed for twenty-four hours at a time, for five days in the week, and for the whole of the forty-eight hours of the remaining two days.

§ 200. The observations were commenced in the early part of April, 1866, and were continued until the 1st of August. It will be seen that occasionally there are days on which no return of quantity of pollen is given. This was generally

---

* If this fluid is intended to be used for the collection of very small and delicate organisms, it will be necessary to exercise great care in preparing it. The spirit should be placed in an ordinary chemical "wash-bottle," or in a bottle from which it can be drawn by means of a syphon. After being allowed to stand some days, three fourths of the spirit should be decanted by means of the tubes in the wash-bottle or by the syphon, so as not to disturb any sediment which may have been deposited, the object being to get rid of all solid matter suspended in the fluid. After the water, glycerine, spirit and carbolic acid have been mixed together, the fluid may be again decanted in the manner described above, and is then ready for use. It is scarcely necessary to say that the mixture should never be allowed to remain open to the atmosphere until placed on the glass.

caused by some accident happening to the slides during the time of exposure; sometimes a high wind with drenching rain would partially wash the pollen away, so that the experiment was not to be depended upon.

For nearly a month after the observations commenced very little pollen was found. On the 30th of May the quantity increased, and was considerably beyond anything that had been collected previously. From this time up to the 1st of August pollen continued to appear on most days whilst the trial was continued.

§ 201. In the first set of experiments the glasses were always placed in a horizontal position, and after being exposed the requisite time each cell—containing about seven hundred microscopic "fields"—was examined separately under the microscope, the number of pollen grains being carefully counted.*

At first sight it would seem to be rather a formidable task to examine daily four slides each having the number of fields named above. If, however, instead of regarding each cell as consisting of seven hundred separate fields we suppose it to consist of a certain number of lines, each line having the width of one field, we simplify the task very much.†

§ 202. The state of the barometer was noted and registered during the greater part of the first course of experiments, but as I did not find that barometrical

---

* For investigations where it is intended to ascertain the exact number of organic bodies deposited in a given space, it is necessary to use a microscope with a stage which traverses by screws, or by racks and pinions. A stage which only allows the slide to be moved by the fingers will be almost useless in such experiments as these.

† When the slide is examined it should be placed in the centre of the microscope stage, so that the line described by working one of the stage screws will be parallel with the line of varnish which forms one side of the cell. By moving the stage slowly from one side of the cell to the other a line, which is one centimètre long and one field in width, will all be brought into view. By moving the stage with the other screw, just the width of a field, another line is brought into view, and may be examined in the same manner as the first. And so the operation may be continued until the whole surface of the cell has been examined. When the quantity of pollen is very great, it is sometimes necessary to use a micrometer with the lines ruled so as to form squares.

variations had any direct action either in increasing or decreasing the quantity of pollen deposited, no attention was paid to this matter in the latter part of the course.

The hygrometrical condition of the air was not ascertained, so that I am not able to say much upon the effect which vapour in the atmosphere has upon the formation of pollen; but although I cannot say exactly what influence a dry or moist condition of the air has upon its formation, I am tolerably certain that a dry state of the atmosphere will cause it to be thrown off more easily when it has been formed than it will be when the air is charged with vapour.

§ 203. In order to try what effect an atmosphere highly charged with vapour would have upon the discharge of pollen the following experiment was tried. A number of ears of rye, after having their stalks inserted in wet earth, were placed under a glass shade so that the air about them might be kept still and be thoroughly charged with vapour. An equal number of plants were treated in a similar manner, but were not placed under a glass shade, and thus were freely exposed to the air of the room in which the experiment was tried. In each case the anthers were quite ripe, the plants being taken from the same part of the field, and, as far as could be seen, were in a similar condition. In both cases the plants were excluded from the direct rays of the sun. The temperature of the room ranged from 65° to 70° Fahr.

In the ears which were exposed to the air the anthers began to throw off their pollen freely in the course of a few hours; but in those placed under the shade not a single anther discharged its pollen, although the experiment was continued for some days.

§ 204. The test here was rather severe. In no state of the atmosphere, during the daytime in England, will there be as much vapour present in the air as we had in this case; but, nevertheless, from the result of this experiment and from other observations I have made, I am satisfied that a humid state of the atmosphere will not permit pollen to be thrown off freely, although it is a condition in which growth may go on rapidly if the temperature is high enough.

§ 205. Temperature, as I have previously intimated, had an important though not a direct action in determining the amount of pollen formed and discharged. A small variation did not, *cæteris paribus*, produce a very marked alteration in the quantity deposited; nor did it seem to signify how often the changes occurred, providing these kept within certain limits.

§ 206. The amount of rain had a more important influence than any other single circumstance. It was not, however, necessary that the aggregate amount should be very great. The time over which the fall was distributed was as important as the quantity. Gentle rain, for a few hours at a time, followed by a day or two of sunny weather, was, if the temperature kept moderately high, more favorable to the formation and discharge of a large quantity of pollen than were days of heavy rain followed by a long period of very hot and dry weather.

It is, however, to be remarked that the quantity of pollen is usually very large for some days after the change from wet to dry weather has taken place, but if the heat keeps up very high the supply after a time suddenly lessens, and does not increase again very rapidly unless rain falls within a given time.

§ 207. For some days after pollen began to appear in appreciable quantity the amount was very small, and if the number had remained at this point—if I may judge from the absence of any very perceptible effect in my own case— it is probable that, in the majority of instances, no symptoms which would particularly attract the attention of the patient would be produced. And this leads me to observe that in some parts of the country a similar state of things will be almost a constant condition in the summer time. Lands which are used for pastures and which are kept moderately well cropped scarcely ever give rise to hay-fever, for the reason that the greater part of the grass never arrives at that degree of maturity to permit the formation of pollen. In lands also which are considerably above the sea-level, and where the average temperature may be comparatively low, the growth of grass may go on, but the flowering may be so imperfect that the quantity of pollen which is thrown off will be but small. In such a case hay-fever, if developed at all, will be very mild in character.

§ 208. In the series of curves shown at Table I we see the general rate of increase and decrease, the variations, and the dates on which these occurred. In these it will be seen that at times the number of pollen grains collected suddenly went down from a high point to a very low one. Until I found that such variations did occur I was never fully able to account for the alteration in the intensity of the symptoms which I often noticed during the hay season in my own case. In the earlier years of my attacks I was inclined to attribute the amelioration to the action of the remedy I happened to be using at the time. I am now satisfied that the remedies used had little or nothing to do with these alterations in the intensity of the symptoms.

§ 209. These sudden diminutions in the quantity of pollen, when they occurred in the ascending scale—or on any date between the 28th of May and the 28th of June—, were invariably due to a fall of rain, or to this latter and a fall in the temperature. This remark also holds good with regard to the descending scale, but perhaps not quite to the same extent.

A good example of this is seen in the changes which occurred between the 10th and 12th of June. On the first of these days the temperature was 74° Fahr.* On the 11th the temperature was 66° Fahr., and on the 12th the number of pollen grains had gone down from 285 to 12; but in the time which had elapsed whilst these changes had taken place rain had been falling for twelve hours; chiefly, however, between the 11th and 12th.

Another notable example of the effect produced by a fall of rain and a decrease of temperature is seen in the descending scale. On the 30th of June the temperature was 90° Fahr., and the number of pollen grains collected

* In all cases the temperature in the sun is indicated.

was 650. On the 4th of July the temperature had fallen to 63°, and the number of pollen grains to 10. Rain had fallen during each day, and in the early part of the time it was very heavy.

§ 210. On taking an average for twenty of the days on which the greatest number of pollen grains were deposited we find that whilst the mean quantity for each day was 364·8, the mean temperature for each day was 79·2°.* On twenty days in which there was the smallest deposit the average was 75·75, whilst the average temperature for these days was 71·5° Fahr.

These results would seem to favour the idea that temperature has a direct and independent influence upon the quantity of pollen formed. When we examine more closely, however, we find that this is more apparent than real. As I have before observed, temperature has a very important action in determining the quantity of pollen formed, but there is no fixed relation between the two. In the early part of the course of experiments three of the warmest days, with an average temperature of 74° Fahr., gave a total of fifty pollen grains for the three days. On three of the coolest days the average temperature was 65·3° Fahr., and the entire number of pollen grains collected was eight hundred and fifty-eight—more than seventeen times the number obtained in the warmer days.

§ 211. One fact was particularly noticeable, namely, that the average temperature of the days which comprise the ascending scale was not so high as that of the descending scale. In the first case we have an average of 76° Fahr. for each day. In the second case the mean is 76·5°. The lowest temperature on any day on which pollen was deposited in appreciable quantity was 60°, and as far as the observations altogether seemed to show it would appear that the pollen of many of the meadow-grasses is not readily thrown off at any temperature below this.

§ 212. Although the amount of pollen gathered was always lessened by a fall of rain, this decrease, as might

---

* Taken between the hours of 10 and 12; generally about 11 a.m.

naturally be expected, was generally compensated for soon after the cessation of rain; and this was always the more marked if with the cessation of rain there had been a rise in the temperature.

As a rule the effect of a fall of rain manifested itself at once, and so rapidly was the effect produced that often a fall of five or ten minutes' duration would, for a time, completely clear the air of pollen as well as of every other kind of solid matter. The effect of a change of temperature was, however, generally not seen for some hours after it had occurred, and this was perhaps a little more noticeable in a rise than it was in a fall of temperature.

§ 213. The maximum quantity of pollen—880—as the table of curves shows, was obtained on June 28th. The maximum temperature occurred on June 27th, and was $96°$ Fahr. The quantity of pollen given above is, however, only the mean of the four slides exposed. The highest number was 1260.* The average temperature of three of the days in the earliest part of the course, when the pollen began to manifest its power, was $71·3°$ Fahr. The average of three of the days at the termination of the course, and when the symptoms of hay-fever had all but disappeared, was $73·3°$ Fahr.

The facts given above on the relation of the temperature to the quantity of pollen collected point to the conclusion that, whilst there is a tolerably close connection between the two, quantity is not entirely dependent upon any given temperature. It is in fact probable that whilst there is a certain temperature which may be considered the normal point for the generation of pollen, a certain amount of variation above or below this may occur without perceptibly retarding this process.

§ 214. To a hay-fever patient it signifies little which pollen it is that produces an attack of the disorder so long as it is produced; but it is a matter of some importance to him to know that if he can so regulate his movements as to avoid certain districts during the flowering period of any plant which may be grown in quantity in those districts, he

---

* Equal to 7870 to the square inch.

has a chance of escaping the attacks. And it is still more important for a patient to know that his chance of escape will be much increased if it is shown that the pollen of one order of plants is the principal cause of his suffering.

Before the experiments were tried I, in common with some other authors, had an idea that a fair per-centage of the pollen found in the atmosphere would not be derived from the Graminaceæ. I have found it very difficult to determine the exact proportion. Of the pollens of other orders a large number are easily distinguished from those of the Graminaceæ, but there are some that even when fresh and when placed side by side with grass pollen are not easily distinguished from it. This difficulty is also increased after the pollen grains have been more or less distorted by being soaked in fluid.

§ 215. So far as I could judge from observation fully ninety-five per cent. of all that was collected belonged to the Graminaceæ. It would, however, not be right to assume that because in this district I found so large a proportion of the pollen to come from plants belonging to the last-named order it would be the same in every other district. It is probable that a very different result would be obtained in parts of the country where plants belonging to other orders are largely cultivated.

§ 216. In attempting to place a mathematical value upon the intensity of the symptoms in any disorder we encounter one of the greatest difficulties with which we can have to deal in the study of disease. There is no known method of constructing a scale by which the severity of a malady can be estimated in the same ratio by all physicians. Then, again, the susceptibility to the action of certain morbid agents is probably not often exactly the same in any two individuals, nor yet in the same individual at different times.

In hay-fever, also, as in many other diseases, there are many other factors which go to make up the sum total of those influences which modify the severity of an attack, and unless we know the degree of susceptibility in any case, and are acquainted with the nature and mode of action of these factors, it is impossible to fix an exact value upon a given dose of the morbid agent. The knowledge of the amount of the dose furnishes only part of the data required. The other portion is an unknown quantity.

§ 217. There is, also, another point to which I think it necessary to refer before I pass from this part of the subject. I have, at times, thought that the continued contact with pollen had a tendency to create a certain degree of tolerance for it. Towards the end of a season I have occasionally found that when the quantity of pollen has been moderately large the symptoms of hay-fever have not been correspondingly severe. Of this, however, I cannot feel very certain. At the end of a season I have always been too glad to get quit of the trouble to permit me to think of lengthening my sufferings by trying if I could exhaust the susceptibility by the repeated application of pollen. I can only, therefore, give the above as an impression which has occasionally arisen—not as an ascertained fact.

§ 218. The study of hay-fever is as much affected by the difficulties of which I have spoken as that of any other disease, and in judging of the action of the varying amount of pollen found in the air we shall have to take these, and also other disturbing causes to which I have before alluded, into account.

In all the experiments 1 have tried one fact stands prominently out, namely, that a certain amount of pollen may be present in the air without producing, in me, any appreciable symptoms. Whether other hay-fever patients would, under the same circumstances, be free from the disorder I cannot say, but I am inclined to think that in this respect the degree of susceptibility will vary in different individuals.

§ 219. After the grasses begin to flower—which in this part of the country is generally early in May—pollen may be found in the air up to the end of September, or even later, if the season is mild; and occasionally, when the second crop of grass flowers vigorously, it may for a short time be found in considerable quantity. Under such circumstances I have sometimes had a return of the malady for a short time in the autumn.

If along with a large quantity of hay-grass there is also a large growth of several of the cereals in any district, with patients who are very susceptible to the action of pollen, the symptoms of hay-fever may be felt more or less from May to September. These facts I have no doubt will in many cases reconcile the discrepancies there are in the statements which are made with regard to the duration of the disease.

§ 220. In my own case very slight symptoms have been felt so early as the middle or latter end of May, but those have generally been too slight to attract attention if I had not by experience known what they were the forerunners of. In the year in which the first continuous experiments were made the attack commenced in good earnest on the 8th of June, but in the table of curves pollen is shown to be present from the 28th of May.

In estimating the correspondence there was between the quantity of pollen and the severity of the symptoms, the plan pursued was first to note the number of pollen grains deposited when the disorder began to appear, and then to make the quantity of pollen and the intensity of the symptoms a standard for estimating the probable rise or fall of those of the following day. Thus, in this way each day was made to do duty as a standard for the next. In all cases the day's symptoms were registered before any attempts were made to ascertain the quantity of pollen deposited.

§ 221. In pursuing this plan no exact estimate of the quantity could be formed from the symptoms merely. Nevertheless, a tolerably correct opinion could generally be formed as to whether there had been an increase or diminution in the quantity, and in most cases it was not difficult to say whether the rise or fall had been very marked.

The time spent in the district in which the experiments were made varied. Generally not less than four hours were spent in this district. Sometimes six hours would be passed in the neighbourhood; but as I found that it made very little difference in the severity of the symptoms which—

ever side of the city I happened to be on—providing I was an equal distance from town—it mattered very little where I passed the time* if this was passed in the open air.

§ 222. A few experiments were tried for the purpose of ascertaining what amount of pollen there is in the air of a dwelling house. I found that as a rule there was very little in this situation even when a large quantity was collected in the open air.

In a room which was seldom entered no pollen at all was deposited on a glass which was exposed the usual length of time—twenty-four hours. In other rooms in which the experiment was several times tried, and which were in constant use, the highest number obtained was six. In a room where I purposely kept a quantity of grass in full flower so that it might throw off its pollen, only eight grains were found on the cell after this had been exposed forty-eight hours; and although I was in the room frequently for an hour at a time whilst the pollen was being thrown off, I had no symptoms which could be fairly attributed to its presence. This result I attribute to the fact that in an atmosphere in which the air is perfectly still, and where the direct rays of the sun do not penetrate, the pollen falls to the ground as soon as it escapes from the anther. In the open air, as I shall have to show farther on, a very different state of things exists.

§ 223. The result of these experiments has led me to conclude that the time spent in a house, unless this is situated in the midst of grass lands in the open country is, as a rule, free from the influence of pollen; or at any rate, that this is rarely present in city houses in such quantity as to give rise to a troublesome degree of hay-fever. Except in very rare cases I also doubt the necessity for shutting up patients in a darkened room at any period of the attack; but of this I shall speak farther on.

§ 224. The highest points in the table of curves corresponded tolerably well with the periods of the greatest intensity of the disease. On June 8th, when the symptoms began to be troublesome, the number of pollen grains

* Except under the circumstances named at § 191.

obtained was sixty-seven. The entry for this day in my note-book states that "I had been in the field only a quarter of an hour when a smart attack of sneezing came on. This was followed by one or two others during the day. There was copious discharge of serum from the nostrils, with itching of the eyelids and hard palate for some time after leaving the district." Again, on June 23rd—the highest point but one on the table of curves—I find the following entry:—"The nostrils have been much inflamed all day, and have discharged a large quantity of thin watery serum mixed with puriform mucus. I have also had several violent attacks of sneezing with watering and burning of the eyes during the day; but the heat in the eyes and nostrils with the constant discharge of fluid from the latter are the most distressing symptoms. The Schneiderian membrane has also been much swollen, but not so as to lead to complete occlusion of the nasal passages."

§ 225. On the day on which the highest number of pollen grains was collected the symptoms were in some respects not so severe as might have been expected. This might in part be accounted for by the circumstance that the constant irritation of the mucous membrane of the nares had caused the nasal passages to become completely occluded for the greater part of the day. In this way less pollen was drawn into the nostrils, and, of course, less irritation arose, and as I have found that the mucous membrane of the buccal cavity is much less sensitive to the action of pollen than that of the nares, even when respiration is entirely performed through the oral aperture, less irritation must arise than when the air passes through the nasal apertures. It is not at all improbable that the slight amelioration of the symptoms, which sometimes occurred during the days which comprise the descending scale, may have been due to the same cause.

What the disorder lacked in intensity in one way, however, it quite gained in another. On the day in question the ophthalmic suffering was very severe. The eyelids and conjunctivæ were much swollen. There was a constant discharge of fluid from the eyes, with intense itching and slight burning. The tumid state of the conjunctivæ also gave rise to a slight appearance of chemosis. The nasal apertures remained occluded nearly the whole of the day, and the symptoms taken as a whole gave rise to an amount of discomfort which only those who suffer from hay-fever can fully understand.

§ 226. The lowest points in the scale were not always marked by a decrease in the severity of the suffering which corresponded to the quantity of pollen gathered. If the interval between two high points was not more than two days it seemed not to give the mucous membrane sufficient time to recover from the effect of one before the other was reached. If, however, the interval was longer than two days the effect was very marked. Such an interval occurred between June 14th and June 21st. On June 18th, five days after a high point had been reached, the symptoms were very mild. There was no sneezing nor any irritation of the nostrils or eyes whilst I was on the ground where the instruments were placed, and on the whole I felt as I do when I am becoming convalescent. On the 19th I find the following entry in my note-book :—" Have been more free from symptoms during the last twenty-four hours than at any time since the attack commenced." On the 20th the number of pollen grains, which on the previous day had gone down to seven, rose to one hundred and fifty. With this rise the symptoms began again to be severe, and continued to be so until the highest point was reached.

§ 227. The remarks made above to a large extent hold good with regard to the changes which occurred in the descending scale, but with this difference that after a sudden decline in the severity of the symptoms and the quantity of pollen these never rose again to the same point they had been at before the alteration occurred; and this was always the case notwithstanding that under such circumstances the temperature remained very high at times. On July 11th and 12th, for instance, the temperature was 90° and 94° Fahr., but the number of pollen grains had gone down from the highest point, 880, to 275 and 260 respectively, and the symptoms had correspondingly declined in severity.

The facts I have given above show conclusively that hay-fever is, in my case, due to the presence of pollen in the air and not to heat.

§ 228. In the year 1867 a second set of experiments was tried near to town. This was done in order to ascertain the number of pollen grains that would be deposited on glasses placed in the outskirts of the city, but still within the boundary of one of the most densely populated parts.

The spot in which the instruments were placed was an open space to the south-west of Manchester, about eighty yards long by about eighteen yards wide. This quadrangle was bounded on three sides by buildings three stories high, and on the other side by buildings two stories high.

When the wind came in a north-easterly direction it would have to pass over a dense mass of buildings quite three miles in extent without coming in contact with a single yard of grass land in which pollen could be formed. In the two directions at right angles to this the distance to the open country would be from half a mile to a mile. In the other or south-westerly direction the distance would be about a third of a mile.

§ 229. Though not in the centre of the city the place selected for the experiments was a good example of an average city residence. I have no doubt, however, that if these could have been made nearer the centre of the city the results would have been slightly different, and would have tended to show still more forcibly than they did the great difference there is to a hay-fever patient between a residence in the town and in the country during the hay-season.

In the first set of experiments four glasses were exposed, and the mean of the four taken. In this series only one glass was exposed, and as this was equally open to the air on all sides, the quantity of pollen obtained may be taken to be nearly what was the maximum in the first course. As in the other case, the symptoms were always registered before the slide was examined, and the point at which these first showed themselves was noted; and, as in the former year's experiments, each day was made a standard for that which was to follow.

§ 230. The table of curves (Table II) shows the time at which pollen first began to appear continuously, and it is curious to observe that the day on which the first important rise occurs in the quantity is exactly the same as is shown in Table I. In like manner, too, there is at the beginning a period of twelve days, during which the quantity is very small. The highest point in the scale was, as will be seen by the table, reached on June 23rd, five days earlier than in the year before. On this day I find an entry in my note-book to the following effect:—"I am much more severely affected than I have been on any day since the attack commenced. The eyes are very hot, and itch intensely, and have a slight burning sensation in the anterior part of the eyeballs, as if hot fluid of some kind had been dropped on to them. The nostrils have discharged freely, and I have had several violent attacks of sneezing."

The changes which occurred in this season (1867) were not, as a whole, so sudden, nor yet so great, as those of 1866. In the ascending part of the scale they were very similar in character—making allowance, of course, for the difference in quantity*—but in the descending part of the scale the fall was much more gradual. The character of the symptoms corresponded very closely with these changes. We had first an absence of symptoms up to the point named above; then an increase in the intensity at each rise up to the highest point; then a continued lessening in severity until all symptoms disappeared at the end of July.

§ 231. If we take ten of the days on which the highest number of pollen grains was obtained in 1867, we find the average for each day to be 46·8. If in the same way we take ten of the highest numbers for 1866, we find the average to be 472·5 per day; thus showing that a patient who resides in a large city during the hay season will not need to come in contact with more than one tenth of

* In a few experiments tried this year in the country, the quantity gathered was generally ten times as much as we had in the city, and it will be seen that the proportion I give afterwards will be about the same.

the quantity of pollen he will have to meet with in the country.

These proportions will of course differ according to the size of the town and the character of the country around it, but the experiments given above prove in a very conclusive manner that hay-fever is less severe in a town because pollen is much less abundant.

§ 232. A number of experiments were again tried in 1869 behind my own residence. This is just outside the periphery of the city, and is a half a mile nearer to the open country (where the first observations were made) than the place selected for the second course. Practically it was a sort of midway between the two. Grass was grown and made into hay within a hundred yards; and as I could be on the spot quite fourteen hours out of the twenty four, it seemed to be an excellent opportunity for trying the experiments under conditions which were slightly more favorable for getting exact results than they had been in the former instances.

In the experiments previously tried the slips of glass were placed horizontally, but in these the slide was placed perpendicularly, in the manner shown at figs. 8 and 9. (Plate V.)

§ 233. In these experiments the same rule was observed as in the first course, so far as regards the registering of the symptoms each day before the slide was examined. The results were quite as conclusive as in the first and second course.

I had here an opportunity of being more constantly in the open air, and in close proximity to the instruments, than I had in the first course. This, I think, helped to make the symptoms accord more closely with the quantity of pollen collected than they had done in the first observations. I also found that it enabled me to predicate with more confidence the probable rise or fall in the number of pollen grains on each day.

As I have given the results of the first course of experiments quite fully enough to enable us to see the connection there is between the quantity of pollen and the

PLATE V.

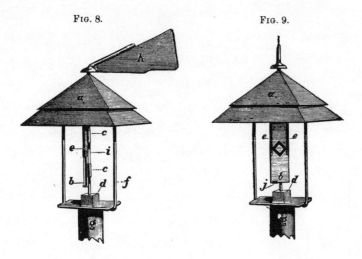

Fig. 8.

Fig. 9.

Fig. 8.—A side view of the instrument represented: *a*, the roof or cover; *b*, an ordinary microscopic slide; *c, c*, sockets through which the central shaft, *i*, passes, and which are soldered to the back of the plate, *e* ; *f*, one of the side pillars, which, with its fellow of the opposite side, supports the roof *a* ; *g*, a socket which fits on to the upper part of a pillar of wood, which, by its lower extremity, is attached to a hinged tripod. By this latter the whole apparatus can be so regulated that the vane, *h*, will have no bias in any one direction, and the slide, *b*, will be exactly perpendicular.

Fig. 9.—A front view of the instrument: *a*, the roof or cover; *b*, a microscopic glass slide, with a cell one square centimètre formed in the centre with black varnish ; *d*, a square hollow pedestal ; *e, e*, clips which turn over the edges of the glass slide and keep this in position. These are attached to the back plate to which the sockets, *c, c* (shown in fig. 8), are soldered ; *g*, a socket which fits on the upper end of a pillar of wood attached to a hinged tripod ; *j*, a spring which is bent forward at right angles to keep the glass slide in position.

Drawn to a scale of $\frac{1}{4}$th.

intensity of the symptoms of hay-fever, it would serve no purpose to enter into the details of this course, and the more especially so as they would not throw much fresh light upon the facts already given. Nevertheless, I must mention one or two matters here to which I have not specially referred before.

§ 234. In addition to those influences which make pollen more or less capable of fulfilling its own proper function in the vegetable world, there also seems to be some influence at work which, independent of quantity and of the condition of the patient, alters its power of producing hay-fever. Whether these alterations are due to one and the same cause I am not at present able to say, but there is no doubt in my own mind that such a cause exists, and that this occasionally alters—so far as hay-fever is concerned—the properties of pollen.

It has also two or three times happened that the slide, instead of having the usual deposit of pollen upon it, has had a quantity of the granular matter spread evenly over the cell; and this has been distributed in such a manner as to preclude the idea that it could have been discharged from the pollen grain after this had been deposited upon the cell. What had been the cause of this mode of distributing the granular matter I was not able to ascertain, but I was certain that it must have floated in the air as free granular matter.

B. *Experiments at high altitudes.*

§ 235. During the second course of experiments my attention was drawn to the circumstance that sometimes when the wind had been blowing right over the city for nearly the whole of the twenty-four hours during which a slide was exposed, there was nevertheless a deposit of pollen. When the wind blew in this direction the nearest point of land where pollen could be formed would be nearly three miles distant; and whatever quantity was deposited at the spot where the instrument was placed, it would have to rise to a considerable altitude and cross the dense mass of buildings which form part of the city and two of the outlying townships of Manchester.

§ 236. Darwin and other observers have shown that dust can be carried very long distances by atmospheric currents,* but this has generally been understood to have occurred when strong winds have carried the dust into the upper atmosphere.† I had at one time the impression that in a quiet state of the atmosphere a very small quantity of solid matter of any kind would be found very high up in the air. It had consequently been a favorite idea with me that if a

---

* In referring to this subject Mr. Darwin says, "I have found no less than fifteen different accounts of dust having fallen on vessels when far out on the Atlantic. From the direction of the wind, whenever it has fallen, and from its always having fallen during those months when the *harmattan* is known to raise clouds of dust high into the atmosphere, we may feel very sure that it all comes from Africa. It is, however, a very singular fact that, although Prof. Ehrenberg knows many species of infusoria peculiar to Africa, he finds none of these in the dust which I sent him: on the other hand, he finds in it two species which hitherto he knows as living only in South America. The dust falls in such quantity as to dirty everything on board, and to hurt people's eyes; vessels have even run on shore owing to the obscurity of the atmosphere. It has often fallen on ships when several hundred, and even more than a thousand miles from the coast of Africa, and at points sixteen hundred miles distant in a north and south direction."—*Journal of Researches in a Voyage Round the World*, by Charles Darwin, F.R.S. London: Murray 1845. 2nd edit.

† In speaking of the cause of whirlwinds, Colonel Reid says:—" It is now a well ascertained fact that whirlpillars are developed in the midst of storms; and being small whirlwinds turning in either direction, they may cause unexpected shifts of wind dangerous to ships." . . . . . "I believe it to be the whirlpillar which carries up volcanic ashes into the upper atmospheric currents in which they are sometimes carried along to great distances." In quoting Redfield on *Aërial Currents*, Colonel Reid says, further:—" We learn from Humboldt that in the great eruption of Jorullo, a volcano of Southern Mexico, which is 2100 feet above the sea, in lat. 18° 45′, long. 161° 30′, the roofs of the houses in Queretaro, more than 150 miles from the volcano, were covered with the volcanic dust. In January, 1835, an eruption took place in the volcano of Cosiguina, on the Pacific Coast of Central America, in lat. 13° N., and having an elevation of 3800 feet, the ashes from which fell on the Island of Jamaica, distant 730 miles N., 60° E., from the volcano. . . . . Few facts in meteorology are more worthy of our attention than the stratiform character of the vast horizontal extension of the aërial currents in different portions of the globe."—*Law of Storms and Variable Winds*. By Lieut.-Col. Wm. Reid, C.B., F.R.S. London: 1849.

patient could, during the hay season, go into a district which lay considerably above the sea-level, he would have a good chance of escaping severe attacks of hay-fever— partly for the reasons given above, and partly because pollen would not be generated so plentifully at high altitudes as at places near the sea-level. Various circumstances, however, subsequently led me to believe that there must be a pretty constant current of air going from the earth's surface to the upper part of the atmosphere, and that this current carried with it a large number of the lighter particles of matter which came within its influence. I was also convinced that this upward current was to some extent independent of those influences which produced movement of the air in the horizontal direction, for the reason that its effects were most observable when little or no wind was blowing.

§ 237. But beyond the interest which attached to the question in its connection with hay-fever, it had a still further interest in the possibility there was of the investigation throwing some little fresh light upon one possible mode of spreading epidemic and contagious diseases. I, therefore, determined to investigate the subject as fully as opportunity would permit.

The problems to be solved were—1st. How high can pollen rise in the atmosphere, and to what distance can it travel? 2nd. What quantity is to be met with in the upper strata of the atmosphere as compared with the lower? 3rd. Supposing pollen to be capable of rising to high altitudes, and of being transported long distances, under what circumstances or by what causes is it made to deposit on the earth's surface? Some of these problems I have partially solved; others there are towards the solution of which I have made little or no approach.

§ 238. Familiarity with the appearance of pollen and its known presence in the atmosphere at certain seasons furnished the means of making comparisons such as do not exist in any other disease. These comparisons had hitherto, however, only been made on the deposits got in the lower strata of air. The question was, by what means should the upper atmosphere be reached by instruments? Two modes presented themselves. One was for the observer to go to some high mountain range, and there to expose the slips of glass in the same manner these had been exposed in the experiments already described. Another method was to send up an instrument by a kite, or by a balloon, in the same district in which the other observations had been made.

§ 239. Against the first plan there were several objections. In the first place, the air on high mountain ranges, such as are accessible to observers in England, might be at best only a mixture of the upper and lower strata. If we suppose a current of air at the earth's surface to pass over a level country and then to meet with a high mountain range, a large portion of the air in this lower current must, in passing, be upraised, and thus we should have a mingling of the upper and lower strata. Then another important objection is that no comparative experiments could be tried at the same spot at a lower level. In most cases there must be a difference of some miles between the base of a mountain range and the apex. And, further, it would in most instances be found that the means of making a comparison—the pollen—would be very scanty in such situations. The only thing that could be done to give any satisfactory results would be to make a course of experiments on the plan I have followed at the lower levels, for two or three seasons, and thus to see if a patient would escape the disorder in such situations. This I have not been able to do, and consequently cannot say positively that a patient would to any extent escape the malady by going into districts considerably above the sea-level. I think it is, however, highly probable that in most instances he would do so, and that in some particular situations the immunity would be almost complete. To the consideration of this I shall return in another chapter.

§ 240. The objections above named induced me to look for some means of accomplishing the object in view which would be free from them, and which would at the same time be easily worked. Partly because of the simplicity of the

PLATE VI.

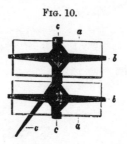

Fig. 10.

Fig. 10.—A front view of the instrument represented. *a, a,* microscopic glass slides with cells one centimètre square (as shown at *d*), formed with black varnish; *b, b,* springs of thin brass attached to the back of the frame, *c, c;* the ends of these springs are turned up at right angles, so as to keep the slides in position; *c, c,* a frame of brass which, at each end, is made to turn over the outside edges of the glass slides in the form of a hook. Another piece which has a similar construction is attached to the centre of the frame and secures the other edges of the slides ; *e,* a tapering brass rod attached to the back of the frame, *c, c.* When the instrument is in use this rod is placed in a socket, which is fastened to the back of the apex of the kite standard, so that the glasses project a little above the kite.

Drawn to a scale of ⅓rd.

plan, and partly because the experiments could be conducted in any district, I determined to try if a kite could be made to carry the apparatus required for the observations. For this purpose I had a kite constructed to carry the instrument shown at fig. 10. (Plate VI.) For the observations made at low levels, to compare with those above, I used the instrument shown at figs. 8 and 9. (Plate V.)

A kite would seem, at first sight, to be a very simple instrument, and capable of being very easily worked; in practice, however, I found it was by no means so easily managed as was first expected, and I found that in order to ensure success it was needful to take every possible precaution. Even when this had been done I had many failures and disappointments. The kite has, however, some advantages over a more cumbrous and costly instrument in the shape of a balloon. It can be used in almost any locality, and with less expenditure of time and money, than would be the case if a balloon were used. In case of accident also it can be replaced at a comparatively trifling cost.*

§ 241. The first experiment at a high altitude was tried on June 17th, 1868. The cells were charged in the usual way with a drop of the prepared fluid. A slide prepared in the same manner was fixed in the instrument shown at figs. 8 and 9, and was placed at the ordinary breathing level. The altitude attained in this first experiment varied from 300 to 500 feet. The day was very hot, and there was during the whole of it scarcely a cloud in the sky. The wind was W.N.W.W., and came from the

* The first kite used was six feet in length by three feet in width, and was made of the usual form, namely, with a central shaft or "standard," and a semicircular top or "bender." In constructing a kite for such experiments as these, the great object should be to attain as high an altitude as possible with as little expenditure of labour and material as may be. In order to accomplish this, lightness, with great strength, are the two principal things to be aimed at. Thin tissue paper was used for covering the kite, but it was found necessary to waterproof this by varnishing it with a mixture of boiled linseed oil and copal varnish. The cord used for raising the kite was also made waterproof by being soaked in a varnish made with paraffin dissolved in paraffin oil.

open country where a large quantity of hay-grass was growing.

I fully expected that pollen would be found in the upper atmosphere, but that it would be in smaller quantity than in the lower. I found, however, in this instance, that the pollen in the upper strata was very largely in excess of that of the lower strata. The number of pollen grains obtained with the lower slide was ten. On the upper slide the number was one hundred and four. I was considerably surprised at this result, and felt sure the slides must have been changed in some accidental way after being taken out of the instruments to be examined under the microscope.

As I had no opportunity of repeating the experiment during the hay-season of 1868 the matter had to stand over until the following year, the impression remaining on my mind that the numbers would be reversed when further trials were made.

§ 242. In 1869 two other experiments were tried, the first of these on July 10th. The altitude attained varied, according to the force of the wind, from 600 to 800 feet. The experiment occupied six hours. The wind blew all the time from the east, and consequently would pass over a large portion of the southern side of the city before it came in contact with the instrument. The nearest grass land would be from two and a half to three miles distant. Five hundred and eighty-four pollen grains were deposited on the upper slide in the six hours. Unfortunately the slide placed on the instrument at the lower level was accidentally damaged before it had been examined, so that I could not make any comparison between the two quantities. A slide exposed, however, for twenty-four hours on the previous day gave only sixteen pollen grains, whilst the one exposed on the following day had sixty-four on it.

The second experiment was tried on July 14th. The weather had been fine for a portion of the day. A tolerably strong wind was blowing from the north-west, consequently this did not come much over the town. No rain had fallen for three or four days. An ascent of four hours— from 3 p.m. to 7 p.m.—gave a deposit on the upper slide of twelve hundred and twenty-seven pollen grains (= 7663 to the square inch), whilst the number obtained at the ordinary level during the same period of time was only eighty.

In 1870 nine other experiments at high altitudes were tried, but five of these only were successful. On April 27th a very small quantity of pollen was found at an elevation of 400 feet, but none at the ordinary level. On May 27th, at an altitude of 1000 feet, forty-six pollen grains were deposited in four hours, whilst the slide at the lower level contained only four. On June 20th an ascent of two hours with an elevation of 600 feet gave four hundred and forty-six pollen grains, but the slide at the lower level, exposed for the same period, gave only thirty. On July 6th, at an altitude of 500 feet, four hundred and thirty-five pollen grains were collected in four and a half hours, whilst the lower slide had only thirty-six deposited upon it.

In an ascent made on August 11th, 1871, the altitude attained was about 1500 feet.* The wind came in a south-westerly direction, and consequently would come right over the centre of the county of Cheshire. The number of pollen grains obtained on the upper slide was fifty-eight, on the lower slide four only.

§ 243. Other observations by means of the kite were

---

* The highest altitude that can be attained with a single kite is about 1000 feet; but this will depend upon the character of the wind. At the suggestion of a friend who assisted me in nearly all the experiments at high altitudes, I tried if one kite could be attached to another after the first had attained a moderate elevation. With a little management and care it was found that the plan was quite practicable. It was by this arrangement that the above altitude was obtained. There is, in fact, no limit to the elevation that may be attained by this method; more than two kites cannot, however, be manipulated very well by the hands alone. If more are sent up a small reel or windlass must be used.

Several other experiments with the two kites were tried, but were unsuccessful. In some of these it was curious to observe the difference there was in the direction of the upper and lower currents of air. In some cases the upper kite would be 15° or 18° (taken horizontally) out of the line formed by the cord of the lower one. The difference in the direction of the two currents must have been considerably more than this, since each kite had a tendency to keep the other in its own line.

made at Filey Bay in 1870. Only one of these was successful. In the former experiments at high altitudes my object was to see what the difference was between the pollen floating in the upper and lower strata of the atmosphere. Here, however, I had a slightly different object in view; I was wishful in this case to ascertain if the upper part of the atmosphere contained any pollen, or any other form of organic matter after passing over about four hundred miles of ocean, and also, if possible, I was wishful to get to know at what altitude it ceased to be present.

It was not entirely on account of the important connection this phase of the subject had with the study of hay-fever that I was wishful to throw a little more light upon it; but partly for the explanation it might help to give of the way in which the causes of disease may be conveyed from one continent to another. Nevertheless, it was not without interest in its connection with hay-fever only. It has already been shown* that dust and volcanic ashes may be deposited in mid-ocean after travelling many hundreds of miles in the upper regions of the atmosphere. There are cases on record in which the attacks of hay-fever have come on whilst the patients have been out at sea, and if it can be shown that pollen will cross large tracts of ocean it is not at all difficult to believe that at times it will descend to the lower part of the atmosphere and be deposited on board any ship that comes in its way. In this manner some of those anomalous cases of hay-fever which have occurred out at sea may be reasonably accounted for.†

§ 244. The instrument shown at figs. 11 and 12 (Plate VII) was devised specially to assist this form of the investigation, and is so constructed that it can be got up to any required altitude before pollen is allowed to come in contact with the squares of thin glass which it is made to carry. It

---

* (§ 236).

† Cattle and sheep are sometimes taken on board ship for use in long voyages, and of course require to be fed. In most cases the food must largely consist of dry hay. In this way also a patient may be thrown in contact with pollen and thus may have hay-fever developed.

PLATE VII.

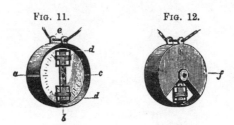

Fig. 11.   Fig. 12.

Fig. 11.—A view of the instrument with the cap f (shown in Fig. 12) removed; a, a case of thin brass in which the wheelwork is placed; b, an arm of thin steel or brass, which is made to fasten on to the pivot shown at its centre. The pieces which project beyond the cross bars at each end are small steel springs, which are turned up at right angles at the ends, so as to keep the squares of thin glass in position. At each end the cross bars are turned over the glass in the form of hooks; c, the dial plate, marked so that each division represents a period of fifteen minutes when the central arm is moving; d, d, squares of thin microscopic glass bordered with black, so that a cell one centimètre square is formed upon them. These cells are charged with the prepared fluid, as in the other experiments; e, small rings attached to the case: through these the piece of cord passes which is attached to the cord used to raise the kite.

Fig. 12.—A view of the instrument with the cap f in the position it is when in use. This latter should be so constructed that it will not sink below the anterior margin of the case, a, as shown by the termination of the dotted line at a.

Drawn to a scale of $\frac{1}{3}$rd.

consists of a thin brass case which contains an arrangement of wheel-work, much like that of an ordinary watch, and driven by a spring in a similar manner.

In the former case the instrument (Fig. 10) was placed at the head of the kite. In this case it was attached to the cord about one hundred feet below the kite. The pivot which carries the arm b was made to revolve once in twelve hours, so that the glass d would be three hours in passing the opening shown in the cap f at fig. 12. By varying the size of this opening the time during which the square of thin glass would be exposed to the wind would vary accordingly. Whatever length of time is necessary to get the kite up to the required altitude before the glass becomes exposed, it is necessary to place the cap f in such a position that the arm will travel that length of time before the glass emerges from under it.

§ 245. The only successful experiment with this instrument was tried at Filey in July, 1870. The wind was blowing from the sea in an easterly direction, and had been blowing, more or less, from the same quarter for twelve or fifteen hours. The altitude attained was nearly one thousand feet. The place selected for the experiment was the narrow slip of land on the cliffs[*] close to the reef rocks,[†] and was as near to the sea as it was possible to get and allow room to work. Grass was growing on the land, but as this was used for pasture and was kept closely cropped by sheep and cattle little or no pollen was formed. The experiment was continued for three hours, and during this time a stiffish sea-breeze was blowing. A glass exposed at the margin of the water showed no pollen or any form of organic matter.[‡] The glass exposed in the instrument at the altitude named above had a deposit of eighty pollen grains upon it.

It would, however, not be right to conclude that pollen or any other form of organic matter would, at certain seasons, always be found at high altitudes in the air which has crossed long stretches of ocean, but this experiment has

[*] The Car Naze.　　　　　　[†] The brig.
[‡] Or any solid matter whatever.

shown that living germs may be carried by the upper atmospheric currents long distances across the sea, whilst the lower strata of air may be perfectly free from them. Thus, one question I had proposed was answered.

If we take an average of the quantities where pollen was present at both levels, we find that whilst the average for the ordinary level was 24 only, for each experiment, that for the high altitudes was 472·33; or in other words, more than nineteen times the quantity was present in the upper strata of air as compared with the lower. Some allowance, however, must be made for the difference there is in the velocity of the air at various altitudes. According to some authorities, this is as *two* for the lower strata to *seven* in the upper,* but even after we have made due allowance for this difference there still remains a great preponderance in favour of the upper strata of air, and it leaves the fact that organic matter is present in such large quantity in the upper regions still unexplained.

§ 246. In some of the experiments slips of ozone test-paper were sent up with the kite. In most cases ozone was altogether absent; in others it was present in small quantity, but never to a higher degree than $2°$ of Schönbein's scale.

In the earlier part of my observations I have entered somewhat extensively into the consideration of the sources from which ozone is derived, and I have there shown that it is present in many situations where hay-fever patients are free from the attacks of the disorder. I had at one time an idea that, possibly, ozone might have the power of altering or controlling the action of pollen in producing hay-fever, especially if this was long subjected to the influence of currents of air which contained a full quantity of ozone. I have, as I have shown, had many opportunities of testing the action of both substances.

---

* In some balloon experiments tried by M. Duprey de Lome during the Franco-German war, the wind in the upper atmosphere blew at the rate of forty-two miles per hour, whilst the anemometer at the Montsaurin Observatory showed a rate of only twelve miles per hour.

Mr. Glaisher had also previously ascertained that ground anemometers do not give nearly the full value of aërial currents.

Pollen has often been tested after it had been for some time subjected to the influence of a sea-breeze which contained a large amount of ozone, but never in any instance have I found this substance to have any tendency to alter the action of pollen.*

§ 247. I have hitherto in these atmospheric experiments confined my attention solely to the consideration of the amount of pollen in the air; it might therefore be imagined by some that this was the only organic matter met with. This, however, would be a great mistake; in no instance in which pollen was present could I say that there were not also germs or spores of some other kind to be found. Generally these were present in much larger quantity than pollen. In many cases the number of spores seemed to be governed by the quantity of pollen, but in other cases there seemed to be no very close connection between the two.

With the form of some of the spores I was tolerably familiar, but there were others which were quite strange to me. It would be foreign to my object to enter here into a description of all that I met with in addition to pollen, and it must suffice, at present, to say that the species were very numerous. The number of spores and germs of all kinds combined was often so great that it was very difficult to form a correct estimate of the quantity.

§ 248. If the advocates of spontaneous generation, who call so persistently for proofs of the existence of large numbers of germs in the air,† will adopt the plan followed

---

* From other experiments I have made with the spores of some of the cryptogams I do not think that, in the quantity usually present in the atmosphere, ozone can lessen the vitality of living germs of any kind.

† M. Pouchet, who was one of the chief advocates of spontaneous generation, said many years ago:—"The imagination is affrighted at the number of eggs and spores which would have to cumber the air to suffice for the universal dissemination assigned to it, but which experience in every way denies."

A later writer (Mr. J. A. Wanklyn), in a letter to the editor of *Nature*, says:—"Great difficulties are involved in the assumption that the atmosphere constitutes a storehouse of germs of all kinds ready to burst out into life on the occurrence of suitable conditions. However small these germs may be, still they must weigh something; and there must be very many of them, seeing that there must be an immense number of kinds of germs, if a volume of air is to supply to any given infusion precisely the right kinds of germs suitable

in these observations, they will have no lack of evidence that they are at times present in very large quantities. In one experiment which lasted about four hours, and in which the number of pollen grains collected at an altitude of 1000 feet, was over twelve hundred, the spores of one of the cryptogams* were so numerous that I could not count them. At a rough estimate, however, there could not have been fewer than six to seven thousand on the slide (= 30,000 to 40,000 to the square inch).

§ 249. There is also another phase of the question which, although it does not strictly belong to the subject, I must not neglect to touch upon before I pass on to other matters. I have shown that, at times, the granular matter of the pollen grain has escaped from the sac before this has been deposited on the slide, thus showing that the former must have floated in the air as free granular matter.

Many of the multitudinous forms of germs and spores which float in the atmosphere have, like pollen, a cellular form, and also—like pollen—have granular contents. If many of these should resemble pollen in its capacity for absorbing water and discharging its granular matter under the influence of moisture, we may have a form of finely divided vegetable and animal matter thrown into the air, which the best modern instruments would fail to discover the origin and nature of, but which might, nevertheless, be a powerful cause of disease. That the granular matter of pollen can and does so act at times I am well satisfied. Such, perhaps, is the state of the active cause of cholera. Of the nature and origin of this latter I do not presume at present to offer an opinion.

§ 250. I must now bring the experimental part of the inquiry into the causes of hay-fever to a close. During its

to the conditions provided by the infusion. Now, chemists are in possession of data showing that the possible amount of organic nitrogenous matter in common clear water and common good air is remarkably small—so small, indeed, that the question may fairly be asked, is it large enough to admit of the requisite number of germs the existence of which the vitalists assume in water and air?" Vide *Nature*, July 21st, 1870.

* Probably they were the spores of the *Ustilago segetum*, or of several species closely resembling these.

course I have shown that pollen of all kinds will give rise to some of the symptoms of hay-fever, and that all the other so-called causes have little or nothing to do with generating the disease. I have also shown that the actual attacks of the disorder, as they occur in the summer, are caused by the pollen which floats in the atmosphere at this time. We have also seen that pollen rises to high altitudes, and is carried very long distances by atmospheric currents; but the most remarkable part of the phenomena exhibited by this course of investigation is the circumstance that there seems to be a zone of atmosphere, commencing some distance above the earth, which contains a much larger number of germs and spores than is found in the lower portion of the atmosphere. How high does this zone extend? How far can germs be carried by the currents which prevail in the upper regions? What is the nature of the force which carries the germs up and keeps them in the higher regions? Under what circumstances do they descend again? Can atmospheric currents convey the active causes of disease from one continent to another? These and many other questions are suggested by the results brought out by these experiments. Future investigations only can answer them. At present the upper atmosphere is almost an unknown region.

CHAPTER V.

ON THE GREATER PREVALENCE OF HAY-FEVER AND ON THE INCREASE OF ITS PREDISPOSING AND EXCITING CAUSES.

§ 251. It would seem that hay-fever has, of late years, been considerably on the increase. It is possible that the fact of my attention having been closely directed to the disorder, for some time past, has brought more cases under my notice than formerly, and that the increase has not really been so marked as it has appeared to me to be. But even if some allowance be made for this probability it will still appear that the disease was less frequently seen fifteen or twenty years ago than it is at the present time. There is no possibility now of determining the exact time at which the disorder first showed itself; but, for reasons which will presently be given, it is probable that it was not only very rare but that it was, in early times, almost, if not entirely, unknown.

§ 252. Every writer on hay-fever has recognised the existence of a peculiar condition of the constitution which gives a proclivity to attacks of the malady. This peculiarity is generally regarded as extremely curious and as one which stands, as it were, outside the pale of those constitutional conditions which give a liability to other forms of disease. Why it should be so regarded is, however, not easy to explain. Probably the yearly recurrence of the disorder and its regular departure at a given time have, more than any other circumstances, led to its being regarded in this light. If its causes had been as inscrutable as those of some of the more fatal disorders and had manifested their power at irregular periods; and, more especially, if death had been the not unfrequent result of an attack we should probably cease to look upon the predisposition as a thing which is out of the usual course.

§ 253. Another point upon which most writers are agreed is the fact of hay-fever being, as has been before stated, a disorder which is almost wholly confined to the educated classes. Some exceptions there may be to this rule, but there can be no doubt that that condition of the nervous system which mental training generates is one which is especially favorable to the development of the disorder; and it is curious to observe that those belonging to, or indirectly connected with, two of the learned professions—theology and medicine—seem to be more liable to it than any other class. Of sixteen patients, whose cases have come more or less directly under my own notice, three are clergymen, three are relatives of clergymen, two are medical men, one is the son of a medical man, two are military officers, one is the wife of a military officer, and three are engaged in mercantile pursuits. The remaining one is the son of a manufacturer, and all may be said to belong strictly to the educated class. Probably when the statistics of the disorder have been more fully and carefully taken these proportions will be somewhat different.

§ 254. One very curious circumstance in connection with hay-fever is that the persons who are most subjected to the action of pollen belong to a class which furnishes the fewest cases of the disorder, namely, the farming class. This remarkable fact may be accounted for in two different ways: it may, on the one hand, be due to the absence of the predisposition which mental culture generates; or, on the other hand, it may be that in this disease there is a possibility of a patient being rendered insusceptible to the action of pollen by continued exposure to its influence. If this latter hypothesis be correct it shows that, in one case at least, the enjoyment of health does not merely depend upon the presence of a high state of vitality, but also, to some extent, upon the acquisition of a certain degree of insusceptibility to the action of the exciting cause of the disease. In this instance I believe that the immunity enjoyed is as much due to the latter influence as it is to the absence of that predisposition which education brings. How then has the disorder arisen, and why has it become more common in these later times? A glance at the state of education and at the condition of the town and rural population five or six hundred years ago, as well as at a few of the changes which have since taken place, may throw some light on the subject and may partially answer these questions.

§ 255. There was a time in the history of this country when education, such as it was, was for the most part confined to the members of the various monastic orders, and even amongst these it was very unequally distributed. With the nobility even learning was not by any means general, and in the class which stood between these and the working classes education was as much the exception as it was the rule, whilst for the latter class it could scarcely be said to have any existence. If, therefore, it is true that the condition which mental training induces acts as a predisponent to attacks of hay-fever we should expect that at this early period this predisposition would be very sparingly developed.

§ 256. But even if we admit the existence of a certain amount of the predisposition in these early times there were other causes at work which would help to make the disease comparatively rare. One of these causes was the smallness of the area of land under cultivation: but not only was there less land under cultivation but upon that which was in use less hay-grass would be raised than is now obtained from the same breadth of land; whilst on some of the land vegetable products of quite another kind were sometimes grown as food for cattle. Buckwheat (*Polygonum fagopyrum*) was one of the plants formerly grown for this purpose in several of the English counties.* Gerarde,

* Some years ago when the branch line of railway was being made between Eccles and Tyldesley (near Manchester), whilst passing a portion of the cutting my attention was drawn to the exceedingly luxuriant growth of the *Polygonum* there was at this spot. Along a portion of the embankment where the soil had

who wrote in the early part of the 17th century, mentions the fact,* and states that buckwheat was not only grown as food for cattle, but in times of scarcity—which in these times were not unfrequent—the seeds were mixed with other grain, and ground and made into bread. The anthers of buckwheat are very much smaller than those of the cereals and most of the grasses; and if this plant was at all extensively cultivated in lieu of the grasses, a much smaller quantity of pollen would be generated than would be formed by the growth of hay-grass on the same breadth of land. Thus, whilst on the one hand, there was a dearth of those influences which lead to a predisposition to hay-fever, there was, on the other, a comparatively small quantity of the exciting cause of the disorder produced.

§ 257. But there were also other influences at work which brought about important changes. Some of these, for a time, checked the development of the disorder, but others not only tended to increase the aggregate quantity of pollen produced at certain seasons, but also caused this increase to occur for the most part in comparatively limited areas. Some of these influences had also the effect of increasing the number of persons susceptible to the action of pollen.

In very early times the cultivation of the soil was the principal occupation of a large portion of the people, but at the same time the ability to take part in the manufacture of some of the simple fabrics then in use was much more general than it is now. The two pursuits were often so blended together that if, for a time, the manufacturing occupation predominated, the individuals so occupied were seldom entirely removed from the influence of a country

been turned up a few months before from a depth of twenty to twenty-five inches, the plants were as closely set as if they had been planted there for some special purpose. It is probable this was a relic of the old Lancashire husbandry, and that in the process of cultivation the seeds had by some chance been buried too deep in the soil to permit them to germinate, and that in this position they must have lain dormant for two or three hundred years.

* *The Herball or General Historie of Plants*, gathered by John Gerarde, of London, Master in Chirurgerie. Very much Enlarged and Amended by Thomas Johnson, Citizen and Apothecarye. London 1633.

life. As time passed on, however, there was a tendency for the various arts and manufactures to be taken up as separate occupations, and for the workers in these to locate themselves in the towns. This tendency had a great impetus given to it in the reign of Edward III. During this reign a number of Flemish weavers, skilled in the manufacture of the finer sorts of woollen cloth, came over and settled in various towns in England, and for greater security the manufacture was principally carried on in walled towns.* But in these times some of the largest towns would not be larger than many of our villages and smallest country towns are now ; and even when the division of labour had been carried so far as to cause a considerable number of the people to be specially devoted to trades and to manufactures, whatever happened to be the nature of their occupation, these would be subject to the atmospheric conditions which prevail in the country to a far greater extent than the inhabitants of our towns are at the present day.

§ 258. After a time the domestic manufacture of woollen cloth as an article of sale began to grow, and it was not unusual for the cultivation of the soil and the manufacture of some kind of woollen cloth to be followed by the same individual. At this period, too, a system sprung up which has continued more or less up to our own time. It was the custom for the clothier, who at that time occupied the place of the mill-owner of the present day, to deliver to the weaver a certain weight of wool to be made into cloth at his own home in the country. This system of domestic manufacture was pretty equally distributed over the whole country. The consequence of all this would be that, with one part of our population the life would be essentially rural whilst with the other, or town population, the condition would, so far as atmospheric influences are concerned, very closely approximate to that of the country manufacturer of a later time.

§ 259. In the early history of the linen, cotton, and silk

* *Wade's History of the Middle and Working Classes.* Edinburgh: W. and R. Chambers, 1842.

manufactures a similar system prevailed. It was at this period not unusual in some of the northern counties of England to see the business of the farmer and small manufacturer combined, and for the workmen employed by the latter to give a helping hand at farming operations at certain seasons if required. As in the case of the woollen manufacture it was quite common for many of the workpeople engaged in the cotton, linen, and silk trades to follow their occupation at their own homes in the country. In these days the click of the shuttle of the hand-loom weaver could be heard almost daily in most of the villages of Lancashire, Yorkshire and parts of Cheshire, as well as in other parts of the country which have since become manufacturing centres. Attached to each cottage there was generally a patch of ground, the cultivation of which furnished occupation to the inmates in their leisure hours and when work was scarce. Now the whole thing is changed. The farmer and the manufacturer have formed two distinct classes, or if the occupation of the former is still retained by the manufacturer it is as a small addition to the business of the latter; and seldom are the workers in one employed in the other. Although the practice of following their occupation at their own homes still lingers among the workpeople in some branches of trade, it is now rarely seen. The hand-loom weaver has almost died out. His place, as well as that of many other outside workers, has been taken by the mill-hand. Thus a large portion of the rural population has been transferred from the country cottage to the mills and workshops of our towns.

§ 260. Whilst these changes have been going on education has been spreading. Not only does it permeate more completely all grades of society, but in every grade it is of a higher quality than in former days. Competitive examinations are now the rule where they were formerly the exception. At all the examining boards in the United Kingdom the standard of excellence has been raised, and there can be no doubt that it now requires a much greater amount of book-learning to reach certain positions in the social scale than it formerly did. Whether all this forcing is an unmixed good is a question I need not enter upon here.

It is true there are parts of the country where some of these changes have not taken place, but these are parts where the population has not increased very rapidly, and which have been, and still remain, purely agricultural; but even here the surplus population has been to a large extent drafted off to feed the ever increasing demand in the large towns, and in this way also a considerable number of individuals have been withdrawn from the preservative influence which a rural or semi-rural life exercises and have been placed under conditions which are favorable to the development of the predisposition to hay-fever.

§ 261. In addition to the spread of that kind of education which consists of regular training and book-learning, there has been a vast advance made in another kind of education; and although this latter is not capable of being formulated or of having its quantity estimated in the way that of the former can be, it is nevertheless of immense value to the country. It is in fact a hidden, but perhaps irregular and somewhat fitful, stream of true technical education which affects, more or less, all below a certain grade in society. The immense progress which has of late years been made in every department of trade and manufacture, and the greater complication and intricacy which have been introduced into these have led to a demand for skilled labour which was not dreamed of in former times. This kind of labour has had, to a large extent, to be formed out of the raw material furnished by the unskilled labourer. In this process of training, faculties, which would otherwise have laid dormant, have been called into play. Intellect of a certain kind has been developed, and, although there may not be many instances of the possession of extraordinary acquirements, there are not wanting examples of remarkable success in various walks of life, amongst those who have had only this irregular kind of training; and there can be no doubt that by this alone the intellectual capacity of the nation has been raised several degrees, and that the constant tendency has been for a certain number of the individuals belonging to this class to be transferred to the educated class, and thus to increase the relative proportion of the latter.

§ 262. Along with all these changes there has been an immense increase in the population of the country at large, and especially in that of nearly all our large towns and cities.* This, combined with the growth of commerce and the general increase of wealth and luxury must have led to a very large demand for the article upon the growth of which the presence of the active cause of hay-fever depends, namely, pollen. These circumstances must not only have led to an increased aggregate production of hay-grass, but also to a large local production. In ordinary times it does not pay to carry hay very long distances, and whatever increase there happens to be in the local demand there must to some extent be an increase in the local production. Thus it must be that in the neighbourhood of all large towns, there will be a greater amount of pollen generated, than will be found in other parts; and in estimating the relative frequency of cases of hay-fever at the present day, it should be borne in mind that this increase occurs for the most part close to the places where a relatively large number of persons susceptible to the influence of pollen are to be found.

§ 263. We have thus seen that at one time the influences which lead to a predisposition to hay-fever were very scanty, and that the production of the exciting cause was at its lowest point. We have also seen that at a later period a large proportion of the population was subjected to the protective influence which a rural occupation seems to afford,

---

* At the close of the 17th century the population of England and Wales was about 5,500,000. London had a population a little over half a million. Manchester at this time contained only 6000 inhabitants, and is said to have had neither printing press nor hackney-coach in it. Leeds had a population of 7000, whilst Sheffield had only 2000 inhabitants.

At the present time the population of England and Wales is nearly 23,000,000. That of London is nearly *ten times* as great as it was in 1700, whilst that of Manchester is *sixty times* as great as it was at the period named. Leeds at the present time contains about 260,000 inhabitants—about *thirty-eight times* the number it had in it in 1700. Sheffield seems to have far exceeded other towns in the rate of its increase. At the present time it contains 240,000 inhabitants—*one hundred and twenty times* the number it had in the year 1700.

and I have shown that large numbers of the people have been transferred from the country to the workshops and mills of the towns, and have thus been placed in circumstances where the predisposition to hay-fever would be most rapidly developed in those who rise to a place amongst the educated class. And lastly, I have shown that the production of the exciting cause has of late years been largely increased.

Taking all these circumstances into account it is highly probable that hay-fever was at one time altogether unknown, and it is tolerably certain that it has not only been much more frequent of late, but that, as population increases and as civilisation and education advance, the disorder will become more common than it is at the present time.

CHAPTER VI.

ON THE SYMPTOMS AND NATURE OF HAY-FEVER.

§ 264. Beyond the circumstance of the predisposition to hay-fever being more common amongst the educated than it is amongst the illiterate, we have scarcely anything to guide us in forming an opinion as to the class of persons, or the kind of individuals, most likely to be affected by the malady. In this respect it does not much differ from many other diseases. If a number of individuals belonging to any class of society were taken promiscuously and examined, it would, without some knowledge of their proclivities, be impossible to say beforehand whether, and to what extent, they would be liable to be affected by any disease with the exciting causes of which they might be brought in contact. It is precisely the same in hay-fever: we have no marks by which the liability to the malady can be recognised, nor do we know of any signs by which the severity of the attacks can be foretold. The disease seems to affect persons of all temperaments and all kinds of constitution, but if there is one temperament which, more than another, predisposes to attacks of hay-fever it is the nervous temperament. Upon this point, however, sufficient evidence to base a conclusive opinion upon has not yet been obtained.

§ 265. Age exercises some influence upon the commencement of the attacks. So far as I am aware there is no instance of the disease having shown itself for the first time after the age of forty. It may, however, begin at a very early age: I have had placed under my care recently a patient who is only four years old, and who had his first attack during the hay season of this year (1872). Generally the malady shows itself later than in this case. According to a table given by Dr. Phœbus,* showing the age at which the disorder commenced in fifty-six cases, one patient only was below six years of age (five years and three months). Out of the entire number eleven were found to have had their first attack when between fifteen and twenty years of age; but although the disorder may come on at any time up to the age of forty, the period between the ages of five and twenty-five years gives a much larger number of cases than the other periods. Out of the total number—fifty-six—thirty-seven of the patients had their first attack in one of the years of the period named. I have already shown (§ 251) that hay-fever is on the increase, and if its causes continue to increase as they have done of late years it is very probable the disease will be seen to commence both earlier and later in life than it hitherto has done.

§ 266. No information that can be relied upon has yet been obtained upon the effect which attacks of other diseases have upon those of hay-fever. In one case a mild attack of gastric fever, attended with congestion of the lungs, seemed to cause the attacks of hay-fever which followed it to be milder in character than they usually were; but, as no experiments on the quantity of pollen in the atmosphere were made at the time, no inference of any value can be drawn from this case. In a certain number of cases patients who suffer from hay-fever are also affected with urticaria, but generally at times of the year when the former is absent. The number of those who do thus suffer is relatively larger than we find in those affected with any other disease. From this it would appear that there was some connection between the two disorders, but as we find that many persons who suffer from urticaria are not affected with hay-fever and that many who are victims to the latter are entirely free from the former, if the connection does exist, it is scarcely probable that it is a very close one; consequently we cannot say that the presence of one disorder is a certain sign of the existence of a tendency to the other. Nevertheless it is not improbable

* *Der Typische Frühsommer Katarrh oder das sogenannte Heufieber Heu-Asthma*, von Philipp Phœbus, M.D., &c., Giessen, 1862, p. 71.

that it may be found that some diseases have considerable influence in preventing or in predisposing to attacks of hay-fever.

§ 267. If the chemical investigation into the nature of pollen had been fully carried out it might possibly help us to form some notion of the general character and scope of the symptoms produced by it; but unless it can be shown that pollen contains some powerful substance of the nature of one of the poisonous alkaloids, or of some other equally powerful class of bodies, the investigation will not help us much. It is in fact probable that, like many other disease-producing substances, pollen is a body with qualities essentially *sui generis*; and that these depend not merely upon the number and nature of the elements which form it, but also upon the mode in which they are combined and upon the relation which the body itself has to the organs whose healthy action it is able to disturb. If this view of the case be correct it is obvious that, as has been before intimated, any investigation which disturbs this mode of combination will alter this relation and may at once destroy the disease producing property of the body.* As, however, no such investigation has yet taken place, we are left to the observation of the effects which pollen produces in attacks of hay-fever and when used in the way of experiment. The question of the vitality of this body has been alluded to before, but need not trouble us here, as our present object is to ascertain the nature and extent of the derangement which it produces, but not to determine the nature of the power which causes that derangement. This may be due to the vitality—or at least may be partly due to it—or may possibly depend upon the presence of some substance which may yet be isolated. The settlement of this question will have to be left to future investigations, but is not without in-

* In a few experiments with the spectroscope, kindly undertaken for me by Mr. Thomas Harrison, of Manchester, two metals—sodium and barium—were found in the pollen of *Lolium perenne*, and also in the pollen of *Secale cereale*. So far as a few experiments of this nature could show, they corroborated the remarks made above on the difficulties that must attend the investigation of the properties of pollen by chemical tests.

terest in the bearing it has upon the study of the nature and mode of action of other causes of disease.

§ 268. First attacks of hay-fever are generally milder and less persistent than they are after a patient has suffered for some years: this is no doubt due to the fact that the susceptibility to the action of pollen is not so marked on its first appearance as it is at a subequent time. There is also in some cases a tendency for the disorder to take on the asthmatic form in later years. In the case of the young patient I have mentioned, although he lives in the country the attack only came on when he was in the midst of a meadow of hay-grass in full bloom. In my own case when the attacks first commenced they were induced only when I was in the immediate neighbourhood of hay-grass in full flower; now it is sufficient for me to be anywhere outside the city to have the symptoms unpleasantly severe at any time during the hay season.

Whether the actual attacks increase the susceptibility or whether this increase is due to other causes cannot at present be determined; but whatever may be the cause there does, in most cases, appear to be a tendency for the susceptibility to become more marked in each succeeding year. It should, however, be borne in mind that, for the reasons already given (§ 262), there must be a continued increase in the quantity of pollen produced and that by making the attacks more severe this may cause an apparent increase in the susceptibility. But even if we make considerable allowance for this circumstance there will still remain an undoubted tendency for the susceptibility to become more marked as time passes on.

§ 269. Dr. Phœbus divides the symptoms into six groups; viz., into the head group; the eye group; the nose group; the throat and mouth group; the chest group; and the general symptoms. Useful as this classification may occasionally be there is, in most cases, no necessity for this minute subdivision. For all practical purposes the simple division into the asthmatic and the catarrhal forms of the disorder will answer quite as well as the elaborate classification given above. If any other arrangement is necessary it would be better to have one which is not only founded on the differences in the structure and function of the parts affected but that would also throw the symptoms into fewer, but at the same time well marked, groups. Such a classification as this would give us four groups; viz.—1st. The symptoms caused by the action of pollen on the mucous membranes of the nares, fauces, and buccal cavity; 2nd. Those caused by its action on the lining membranes of the larynx, trachea and bronchial tubes; 3rd. Those caused by its action on the conjunctiva and the structures adjoining; 4th. General symptoms.

A patient may suffer from one or from all the phases of the disorder, but whatever difference there may be in the symptoms the malady is one and the same and due to the same cause. In a very large number of instances the disease is purely local and whatever may be the function of the part affected we shall find that we generally have one special morbid condition present and that this condition in each case gives a peculiar character to the symptoms. Whatever classification we adopt, the symptoms will tend to form themselves into the two groups spoken of above, and will exhibit themselves in this way to the eye of a casual observer. In one form of the disorder—the catarrhal form—we have not much pain and scarcely any dangerous symptoms. In the other, or asthmatic form, though there is very little actual pain, the distress and suffering is often very great and frequently the attacks appear to be very dangerous.

§ 270. Hay-fever is said by some writers to have premonitory symptoms: these are said to consist of a feeling of weakness, languor, repugnance to food, coated-tongue, constipation alternating with diarrhœa, sleeplessness, irritability of temper, and a feeling of exhaustion when the weather is hot.

Dr. Phœbus gives three stages of the disorder:—1st. The stage of development; 2nd. The paroxysmal stage; and 3rd. The stage of convalescence. In speaking of the first he does not seem to view it as a true premonitory stage; "it lasts" he says "only a few days at most" and as a rule even a less time than this: sometimes not more than an hour elapses before the paroxysm shows itself, and in some cases the latter comes on at once. In one case which Dr. Phœbus mentions the attack came on immediately when bunches of ripe grass and wild flowers were brought to the patient by some friends.

If there are premonitory symptoms in hay-fever these must be produced in one of two ways, namely, either by the causes of the disorder itself or by causes which have no necessary connection with it. If produced by the former they must be of the same nature as those of the acute stage of the disorder, differing only in degree. But if produced by the latter they may be more or less different in character, and since they may thus differ and are produced by unlike causes they cannot be a necessary and invariable antecedent to attacks of the genuine disease.

§ 271. This view of the case is supported by the fact that the malady can, by the application of the requisite quantity of pollen, be brought on at any time without the development of premonitory symptoms; and especially by the fact that however often and however slowly or rapidly these artificial attacks may be produced they are never preceded by symptoms such as have been spoken of. In the case mentioned by Dr. Phœbus the attack came on suddenly and without any such symptoms. I have, as has been stated, several times had similar attacks when brought suddenly into contact with pollen, and there are scattered through the works of writers on hay-fever records of many similar cases. But in order to test the matter more fully a series of observations was made on the temperature and on the pulse of a hay-fever patient during two months of the year 1867. The observations were commenced on the 28th of April—six weeks before the attacks of hay-fever usually came on—and were continued to June 28th, this being the period at which the quantity of pollen collected was generally at its highest point, and, as a matter of course, the time at which the attacks were also at their highest degree of intensity. The time was divided into two equal periods, viz., one comprising the days occurring between the 28th of

April and the 28th of May, and the other those between the 28th of May and the 28th of June. In the first period we have generally, in this part of the country, no symptoms of hay-fever showing themselves. In the second, the disorder commences and goes on from its lowest to its highest point. The average temperature observed during the first period was 97·0° the maximum being 98·0° and the minimum 95·4°. In the second period the average temperature was 97·4°, the maximum being exactly the same as in the first period, viz., 98·0°, whilst the minimum was 95·7°. In all cases the temperature was obtained by placing the thermometer in the axilla. The pulse varied relatively almost as little as the temperature. In the first period the average was 70·22 beats per minute; the maximum being 78, and the minimum 60. In the second period the average was 68·8, the maximum 78, and the minimum 64. These experiments along with the facts previously given show that in some cases, at least, there are no premonitory symptoms, and that these cannot therefore be a condition essential to the proper development of hay-fever. I have, as I have stated above, watched the development of the disease in my own case and also in the cases of the patients I have had under my care, and in no instance have I seen it to be preceded by phenomena such as those referred to at § 270.

§ 272. In some few cases, however, premonitory symptoms may be seen, but only in a few. From the time that pollen first comes in contact with the mucous membranes of a patient, during the ordinary attacks of the disorder, there must be some action going on, but it is not certain that this can be perceived by the patient in all cases. In my own case I found that if the deposit on the glass slide (§ 192) did not amount to more than an average of ten pollen grains in the twenty-four hours, the disturbance in the action of the mucous membranes was not perceptible to me. In some instances I do not doubt that the insusceptibility may reach a much higher point. Probably in these cases a portion of the deposit is rapidly thrown off, just as other foreign matters are, and that up to a certain quantity the membranes are able to tolerate its presence without their action being in any way disturbed, but once let this point be passed and we have all the phenomena of direct and reflex action exhibited which pollen is capable of producing.

In some cases, however, it is probable that, after the pollen grain has burst in the manner described at § 147, a portion of the granular matter makes its way through the walls of the capillaries into the blood current, but just as we find a certain degree of tolerance for the action of pollen when in contact with the mucous membranes, so we may have a similar degree of tolerance for the presence of the granular matter in the blood. Then again I believe that not only the power of resistance varies in different individuals, but that the power of elimination also varies. In some cases the granular matter may be thrown out of the circulation quite as quickly as it enters, and so long as this is the case no symptoms can be noticed; but where the power of elimination does not equal the rate of absorption, an accumulation must take place and, sooner or later, constitutional disturbance must be set up; and this disturbance may, in some cases, be seen before any local symptoms have been manifested. In this way premonitory symptoms and a stage of development may be produced, but if by the latter term any such action, as that which occurs during the period of incubation in zymotic diseases, is to be understood, we must refuse to accept the definition because it has never yet been shown that pollen has any of the properties of a ferment. As I have before observed the premonitory stage will be seen in very few cases; why it should not be seen in all it is not possible to say, any more than it is to say why the exciting causes of other diseases do not affect all who suffer from them in the same way and to the same extent.

§ 273. In most cases, and especially in the earlier years of the disease, the action of pollen seems to concentrate mostly in the nasal passages; next to these come the eyes, then the buccal cavity and the fauces, and lastly, the larynx, trachea, and bronchial tubes. This order is, however, subject to much variation in different patients, and although the symptoms brought on by the affection of the parts last named are often very prominent, and apparently very dangerous, it is, as I shall be able to show, not because of the greater amount of irritation set up in the parts, but because of the importance of the function which they discharge.

The first symptom of the presence of pollen is generally itching of the parts with which it is first brought in contact. This is sometimes so mild as scarcely to be perceptible, but it may go on to a degree which is very severe, and which has more or less of a burning feeling with it. Generally the irritation is first felt in the hard palate and the fauces, then in the nostrils, and lastly in the eyes and face. If the wind is moderately strong the irritation may be felt in the eyes before any other part has become affected; and if the wind is at all cool the patient may imagine that this latter has been the principal cause of the derangement, whereas it is mainly due to the extra quantity of pollen which the increased velocity of the wind brings into contact with the conjunctiva.

When once the production of pollen has, during the hay-season, passed beyond a certain point the quantity may increase so rapidly that in twenty-four hours, or even in less time, the attack may pass from its most incipient condition to the true catarrhal stage. This is characterised by the discharge of thin watery serum from the nostrils, by violent attacks of sneezing, and in some cases by a tendency to lachrymation. Generally the violent attacks of sneezing precede the discharge from the nostrils, but the coryza may be the first symptom of an attack. In the earliest stage of the disorder the fits of sneezing are not very long or very severe, but when the malady has become fully developed they become so violent and seem to take such entire possession of the patient, when they do come on, that, for the time being, he loses all control over himself. In some cases the patient will sneeze twenty or thirty times in succession, and whatever he may be occupied with when the fit comes on he is obliged to set it aside and resign himself to the paroxysm until it is over.

§ 274. After the attack has lasted for a short time the submucous tissue in the nasal passages begins to swell, and if the quantity of pollen in the air becomes moderately large this will go on increasing so rapidly that in a short time no air whatever can be drawn through the nostrils. This swelling and stoppage in the nares often alters in a very curious and apparently unaccountable manner. After both passages have been equally closed for a time, if the patient gets into a recumbent position, so as to lie on one side, the nasal passage which is uppermost becomes after a short time quite open, whilst the lower one becomes still more completely occluded. This change is caused by the fluid in the submucous tissue gravitating towards the lowest part, and as often as the position is changed this alteration in the condition of the two passages will take place.

During the hay season most patients not only have paroxysms of sneezing in the day, but frequently also during the night, and especially when the disorder is just arriving at its highest point of intensity. I have myself had such attacks often, and knowing that pollen was seldom present in the air of a bedroom in quantity sufficient to bring them on, I was not able to account for them. After some time, however, I noticed that these attacks only came on when the nasal passages had been more or less occluded for a time, and that so long as there was no change in the condition of the two when they were swollen, the sneezing in the night did not occur by any means so often as it did when one of the nares suddenly became permeable to air. On trying the experiment I found that the paroxysms of sneezing could be brought on by changing from side to side whilst in the recumbent posture, so as to give time for the fluid in the submucous tissue to gravitate and close the lower passage whilst the upper one became patent. It seems as if the sensibility of the Schneiderian membrane becomes lessened by the pressure of the fluid, and as soon as this pressure is removed by the gravitation of the fluid, not only does the normal amount of sensibility return, but for a short time some degree of hyperæsthesia is acquired. In this way some of the violent attacks of sneezing which occur in the night may be accounted for. Whether this is the true explanation or not it is quite certain that in most cases pollen is not present in sufficient quantity to bring on an attack, and as there is neither light nor any other presumed cause of hay-fever present, the explanation here given seems to be the most reasonable. But there are other important symptoms which this change in the position of the effused fluid will help to account for. To the consideration of these I shall return presently.

§ 275. So long as the supply of pollen is kept up the sneezing and discharge of serum continue, but the frequency and severity of these do not in all stages of the disease entirely depend upon the quantity of pollen inhaled. The degree of occlusion in the nasal passages varies in the day as well as in the night, but not to the same extent. If the occlusion has been tolerably complete in one or both nostrils for some hours, and by any chance suddenly lessens, the patient may have a violent attack of sneezing, notwithstanding that he may be inhaling a very small quantity of pollen at the time. If the average quantity is large, however, the swelling of the submucous tissue continues—subject to the variations above alluded to—the alæ nasi, as well as the lining membrane of the nares, become tender and inflamed, and have a tendency to bleed slightly if rubbed. The patient frequently finds that air can only be drawn through the oral aperture, and if he sleeps he finds on awaking that the tongue and the whole buccal cavity are more or less parched. As the disorder progresses the discharge from the nostrils becomes more inspissated and puriform, especially early in a morning. This I found to be more marked in the descending scales, shown in Tables I and II, than in the ascending scales. Occasionally, in the latter stages of the disorder the puriform mucus is slightly tinged with blood, and thus gives to the discharge something of the colour of the sputa of pneumonia in the latter stages of this disorder.

§ 276. After the disease has lasted some three or four weeks—varying in time according to the kind of season and the susceptibility of the patient—it begins to decline. If the season is a very favorable one for hay-making it will decline rapidly, and this, as every one knows, is generally the most favorable with a very high temperature. When any of the cereals happen to be in bloom at the time hay-making is about finishing in any district, patients residing in this district will find their attacks to be prolonged, and if it happens that a second crop of grass comes into flower before the harvest has got over, the attack may seem almost continuous from May to September.

When once the stage of convalescence has set in, if the patient keeps free from the influence of pollen, the recovery is very rapid. This may, however, appear to set in two or three times in the course of a season. If there is a fall of rain for three or four days in succession, and especially if this is tolerably continuous, the symptoms moderate so quickly that the patient may think the stage of convalescence has commenced. Unless the hay has been got in, however, he may generally expect a return of the disorder before the season is over. When the patient does get fairly from under the influence of pollen, however, the change is very marked. A single night is sufficient to produce a very agreeable change. However profuse the discharge from the nostrils may have been, it rapidly lessens and becomes more inspissated and puriform. The swelling of the submucous tissue subsides, the heat and tenderness of the alæ nasi and of the lining membrane of the nares lessens, and in the course of three or four days the patient considers himself quite well. Generally, however, the convalescence is much more slow than this, for the reason that in most seasons the quantity of pollen diminishes slowly. So much depends upon accidental circumstances that no rule can be laid down. A rapid growth of hay-grass with a very favorable hay-making season will make a short—though it may be sharp—attack, and *vice versâ*.

§ 277. If active exercise is taken when the disorder has become fully established the irritation in the hard palate, the nostrils, and the fauces will become very marked. The fits of sneezing also will become more violent and prolonged. When we remember that the quantity of air inhaled in violent exercise is three to four times the quantity we take in in a state of rest, it is easy to see that rest and exercise must make a wide difference in the severity of the symptoms. Many patients have thought that exposure to the heat of the sun has made their attacks more severe, but the real reason has been that whilst they have been taking active exercise in the open air they have been inhaling a much larger quantity of pollen than they would have inhaled in a state of rest. It was for this reason that Bostock had the symptoms more severely developed whenever he ventured into the open air whilst residing at Ramsgate.

Dr. Phœbus notices that exercise—especially that of a fatiguing nature—causes exacerbations, but this he says is often " only by causing the patients to be heated or rather by getting cold after being heated." The great difference between the amount of air inspired in a state of rest and during active exercise seems here to be completely lost sight of, as are also other important facts. Active exercise, if indulged in for any length of time, is generally taken in the open air, whilst rest is usually taken in a house, and I have shown that the quantity of pollen in the air of an ordinary dwelling house is as a rule very small, whilst that in the open air may be very large.

At the commencement of an attack of hay-fever the difference between the amounts of the pollen inhaled under the two conditions will not be very marked, but when the disorder is getting near to its height the difference in the gross quantity is, as will be seen by the results of the following experiments, very great.

§ 278. In these observations the instrument shown at Figs 3, 4, and 5 (Plates II and III) was used. Three trials were made at different periods of the day: in the first trial 500 inspirations, made in thirty minutes, whilst the operator was perfectly still, gave a deposit of 115 pollen grains on a space of one square centimètre. During the same time thirty pollen grains were deposited on the glass placed in the instrument shown at Figs. 8 and 9. In another experiment, in which the operator was walking at the rate of two miles per hour, 500 inspirations gave 140 pollen grains; whilst in the same space of time twenty-eight were collected on the glass placed on the vane (Figs. 8 and 9).

In the third experiment 1000 inspirations, made whilst the patient was walking at the rate of three miles per hour, gave a deposit of 253 pollen grains. During the same time the glass placed on the vane gave fifty-eight only.

In these three experiments we have a total of 508 pollen grains obtained by 2000 inspirations: in these the air was made to pass over a space of one square centimètre of the prepared glass at a rate varying from seventeen to twenty-eight respirations per minute, each inspiration taking in from thirty to forty cubic inches of air. The total of the deposits obtained on the slides placed on the vane was 115. Comparing these quantities we find that we have 4·4 pollen grains inhaled for each one that is deposited on the glass.

§ 279. If we institute a similar comparison to that made in the deposits obtained in the ordinary way, we find, in this case, that the difference between the quantity of pollen inhaled whilst in a state of rest, and during violent exercise, is very considerable. Ten hours passed in the open air in a state of rest would give a deposit of 2300 pollen grains; but if we suppose that three times the quantity would be inhaled during violent exercise the number would be 6900; or in other words we should have an extra deposit of 4600 on the same space of mucous membrane. This number is rarely, if in any case, reached, because it seldom happens that a patient passes ten hours consecutively in the open air, and very rarely does it come to pass that violent exercise is taken for so long a period. In proportion, however, to the amount of exercise taken and the length of time passed in the open air during the period the grasses are in flower, so will be the approach to the results here given; and if we make an exact estimate of the difference between the number of respirations and the volume of air taken into the lungs, during active exercise and in a state of rest, we shall find that the percentage of increase given above, large as it is, will be rather under than over the mark. The inevitable consequence of this must be that exercise in the open air must, during the hay-season, increase the severity of the attacks of hay-fever.

§ 280. The mucous membranes of the fauces and of the

buccal cavity do not seem to be so sensitive to the action of pollen as that of the nares. This may, however, be more apparent than real. If swelling of the submucous tissue does occur, it will not be so much seen on account of the structures being soft and yielding; and if fluid is thrown off by the mucus follicles, this will be much diluted by the ordinary glandular secretions of the buccal cavity, and will be rapidly carried off. Nevertheless some degree of congestion of the mucous membrane and swelling of submucous tissue do occur, but not by any means to the extent they do in the nares.

The symptoms caused by the contact of pollen with the lining membrane of the pharynx are itching and slight burning or pricking; with these there is sometimes a sensation as if there was a thin film of some delicate substance stretched across the pharynx in places. Occasionally there is a little hoarseness, but this is not often present. The itching is generally felt to be very severe in the upper part of the pharynx and in the Eustachian tubes; and not unfrequently it extends to the meatus externus. Sometimes there is slight dulness of hearing, but this may be so slight that the patient will scarcely notice it unless his attention is specially drawn to the circumstance. Deglutition is very rarely interfered with, but there is occasionally a sense of dryness and obstruction in the throat on awaking in a morning.

If we examine the throat in the earliest stage of the disease very little change will be seen, but later on there may be redness and swelling of the mucous membrane. There is also in the daytime a little extra secretion going on, and especially when the attack is getting near to its highest point of intensity; but, as I have before intimated, this is so intermixed with the ordinary glandular secretions that it is difficult to arrive at any precise notion of its quantity or its character. And on account of the tendency there is for the effusion in the submucous tissue to diffuse itself, it is not easy to distinguish it or to say whether it is much or little. The throat symptoms, like those of the buccal cavity, to which indeed they really belong, vary much in intensity in different individuals; they may in a few cases be somewhat severe, but generally they will be very mild.

§ 281. When pollen is brought into contact with the eye the phenomena exhibited are very marked, and in one of its symptoms very characteristic of its mode of action. Generally, however, these show themselves later than the other symptoms do; the reason for this I shall refer to presently.

In addition to phenomena of a purely physiological character we have also some which are due to mechanical irritation. Whilst the quantity of pollen is small the ordinary fluid secretions of the eye will be sufficient to clear it away by the natural channel—the nasal duct—just as they do other foreign matters deposited by the atmosphere. When, however, the quantity of pollen becomes large it will not be so readily cleared away, and a portion will get between the ocular and palpebral layers of the conjunctiva, and thus severe irritation may be set up; and this will be all the more likely to be the case after the patient has been out in a tolerably strong wind during the height of the hay-season. The difference between the quantity of pollen inhaled and that which is thrown against the eyeball by the force of the wind, may be judged of by the results of the experiments just quoted. In one sense it is a fortunate thing for the patient that this difference does exist, for if the same quantity of pollen that is inhaled came in contact with the eyeball his condition would be almost unbearable. This difference will, however, account for the fact that the eye symptoms are generally later in showing themselves than are the nasal symptoms.

§ 282. In the eyes, as in the other regions, the first symptom of a commencing attack is itching. At first it is very mild, but as the hay-season progresses it is more distinctly felt and soon becomes very troublesome, and is frequently attended by a slight burning sensation, which extends to the deeper parts of the eyeball. When the disease is fully developed the lachrymal canals and nasal ducts become almost entirely closed by the swelling of their submucous tissue, but I have never been able to decide whether the irritation which causes this occlusion commences above or below, or, in other words, whether it is caused by the pollen which passes down the nasal duct from the eyeball, or by that which is deposited in the nostril in the process of respiration. It is, however, probable that both causes operate to produce the effect, and it is also probable that some portion of the derangement is due to the reflex action of the irritation which is set up in the nasal passages. At whichever point it commences the effect is the same, namely, a partial or total occlusion of the nasal ducts, and, as a consequence of this, a constant tendency to lachrymation; but there is no doubt that the secretion of the lachrymal gland is also increased by the presence of pollen on the surface of the eyeball.

§ 283. A short time after pollen first comes in contact with the eye the conjunctival vessels become injected, and generally the larger capillaries show the first, but occasionally when the patient has been much exposed to the wind whilst the quantity of pollen in the air is large, the anterior surface of the eyeball may be covered with a pale crimson or pink tinge from congestion of the smallest capillaries. After a time the itching and burning become so troublesome that the patient finds it difficult to resist the temptation to be constantly rubbing the eyes, but the relief this gives is very transient and, in the end, adds much to the irritation. Occasionally shooting pains of a neuralgic character are felt in the back part of the orbit and in the eyeball, and when the attack has been very severe or long continued slight chemosis may be seen; generally, however, this latter symptom will only be seen in certain cases, and then only when the quantity of pollen in the air is at its maximum. In very severe attacks also the eyelids become œdematous, and this is often more observable in a morning than it is in the latter part of the day, but in some cases this condition will be seen at all parts of the day.

§ 284. When the disorder has lasted some time there is often a little photophobia present, and this may be sufficiently severe to cause the patient to seek the shade rather than the broad sunlight. In my own case, however, I have never found it necessary to remain in a darkened room or even to avoid a moderate degree of sunlight. Even after being exposed to the action of pollen and strong sunlight for six or eight hours in the day, and when, as a consequence, the conjunctivæ have been very much congested, I have frequently worked at the microscope for two or three hours in the evening without causing any additional irritation or inconvenience. In this case as in every other I found that if I could get beyond the reach of pollen the symptoms, whatever they were, were sure to improve. I have also in my own case sometimes thought that for a short period at the height of the disorder the sight has been obscured as if from an alteration in the normal convexity of the cornea, but when tested by placing small print before the eyes I have never been able to discover any marked alteration in the focal distance at the time the test has been used.

§ 285. The eyeball and its appendages seem to be as sensitive to the action of pollen as is any organ with which it comes into contact, and if the irritation in the eye were to be kept up by a large quantity of pollen being constantly applied, it is highly probable that mischief to the deeper seated structures would be the result; but what would be the nature and extent of the derangement it is not possible at present to say. In ordinary attacks of hay-fever the mischief seems not to extend beyond the subconjunctival cellular tissue. In no case have I ever seen any sign of effusion between the layers of the cornea, nor have I ever seen the sclerotic coat to be affected; although I think it is quite possible that it may be in some cases.

The discharge which comes from the eye, like that which comes from the nostrils, is at first thin and watery, and no doubt largely consists of the secretion of the lachrymal gland. After a time, however, it becomes more inspissated; and although it rarely happens that it contains any considerable quantity of pus, this may sometimes be the case; and often when the effused fluid seems to the naked eye to be tolerably transparent, by the aid of the microscope pus-cells may be detected in it.

§ 286. When once the quantity of pollen in the air has got to its maximum and begins to decline, a very marked change in the condition of the eye will soon be seen. The improvement will not, however, always be steady and gradual; but like all the other symptoms of hay-fever will be influenced by the sudden changes in the quantity of pollen. There will at times be a rapid improvement; the congestion of the conjunctival vessels will quickly lessen; the itching and burning will subside and the œdema of the eyelids will disappear. Often, however, the patient, who thinks he is becoming rapidly convalescent, finds that, after a few days of improvement, a relapse comes on; but there is this peculiarity in the attacks which occur in the latter part of the season (from the latter end of June to the beginning of August*), namely, that they rarely attain to the same degree of severity they have in what I call the ascending part of the scale.

§ 287. The last symptoms to disappear are the œdema of the eyelids and the chemosis (when present); but the changes above alluded to do not take place in the same order nor in the same time in all cases, but after the patient gets entirely from under the influence of pollen the improvement will be comparatively rapid. The experiment cited at § 136 shows that even after the disturbance had been much more severe than it is in an ordinary attack of hay-fever the congestion had almost disappeared at the end of eighteen hours, and that after thirty-six hours had elapsed all traces of the derangement were gone. A single night, even in the height of the disease, will in most cases bring about some improvement, for the simple reason that during the night time the patient does not come in contact with pollen, and in this way it may seem to some that the disease has somewhat of a remittent character. Taking the eye symptoms as a whole I believe they disappear rather sooner

* This remark applies, of course, only to the part of the country where my experiments have been made: more south the time will be earlier, and more north later.

than the nasal symptoms; that is to say, the nasal mucous membrane is longer in recovering its healthy condition than the conjunctiva is, but in this respect as well as in others there will be some little difference in different cases.

§ 288. Dr. Phœbus and other writers speak of very decided head symptoms which the former places in a separate group. So far as I have observed, there are few symptoms of this kind which cannot be referred to one of the other groups. There are occasionally shooting pains in the head, but I think these are, in character, closely allied to the neuralgic pains I have mentioned as occurring in the eyeball and orbit. I have never seen any symptoms which had the appearance of being caused by congestion of the meninges of the brain or of the brain substance. There is in some cases a considerable amount of tinnitus aurium: what the exact cause of this is I have never been able clearly to make out; but I do not think it is caused by derangement of any part of the nerve centres. It is probably due to irritation of some portion of the tympanum or membrana tympani, or possibly to reflex action. The neuralgic symptoms commonly depart with the other symptoms, but the tinnitus may remain for some weeks or even months.

§ 289. The asthmatic symptoms of hay-fever are by far the most important of any of the groups because they are the most troublesome and the most dangerous. Like all the other derangements caused by pollen, they vary in intensity in different individuals and in different seasons. In some cases there is only a very slight sense of obstruction in the breathing; in others the derangement may cause great suffering and at times may seem to endanger life. The symptoms are, as I think I shall be able to show, due to the obstruction caused by the altered condition of the submucous cellular tissue of the larynx, trachea and bronchial tubes, for effusion into the connective tissue of any one of these will give rise to the asthmatic symptoms, and it is exceedingly difficult to decide which has the greatest share in producing these.

In many of its symptoms hay-asthma closely resembles

ordinary asthma, and unless we know the exact history of the case we may be investigating, we shall find it always difficult and sometimes impossible to decide which species the case belongs to. In both there is the same sense of tightness across the breast at the commencement, and as the disease advances there is the same loud wheezing and slow inspiration and expiration. There is also at first dry cough or cough with scanty expectoration in both forms of the disorder, and as the breathing becomes more and more difficult the face may be pale and anxious looking. If the dyspnœa still increases, in both phases of the disorder the face will become livid and turgid, the patient will seem as if threatened with suffocation, and will try to fix himself in such a position that the respiratory muscles can act with the greatest vigour, and this will almost invariably be in the upright position, with the arms and hands firmly fixed on some article of furniture. In both cases too the voiding of a thin frothy sputum may be one of the first signs of approaching relief, but this latter is not so much the case in hay-asthma as it is in ordinary asthma.

§ 290. There are, however, some points in which the two disorders differ, and which it is important for us to notice. In ordinary asthma the attack usually comes on in the night, and is often preceded by a long-continued fit of dyspepsia. In hay-asthma the first attack of the season generally comes on in the daytime, and although disorder of the stomach may be present and may help to make the malady more severe when it does come on, it is usually quite independent of dyspepsia. In hay-asthma the attack may and often does come on in the open air, but in ordinary asthma it generally comes on in the house. In the one case the occurrence of the disease is entirely dependent upon the inhalation of pollen; in the other it is, so far as we know at present, entirely independent of it. And again, unless the patient is brought accidentally into contact with pollen, hay-asthma only comes on during the hay-season, whilst ordinary asthma may come on at any time of the year and is most common in winter.

There is also another important difference between the

two forms of the disorder. In ordinary asthma there are paroxysms with intervals of perfect freedom, at least in the early and less confirmed state. In hay-asthma this scarcely ever occurs in so marked a degree as in ordinary asthma; there may be remissions and sometimes even distinct intermissions for short periods, but the tendency is for the disorder to continue with more or less severity during the whole of the hay-season. And lastly, if coryza does accompany an attack of common asthma it is rarely as severe as it is in hay-asthma, and we scarcely ever see the conjunctivæ affected as they are in the latter disorder.

§ 291. In some instances the coryza and eye symptoms may show themselves before any difficulty of breathing is noticed, but occasionally the reverse may be the case; frequently, however, they will come on together. The first symptom of an asthmatic attack will most commonly be the sense of tightness and weight across the chest of which I have previously spoken. In most cases the cough will at first be dry, or if there is expectoration this will be but scanty. In some few instances, however, it may be copious from the commencement, and if this is the case the dyspnœa does not generally become so severe as it is when the expectoration is scanty.

In the early stage of the disorder the difficulty of breathing is not very great, and if the patient lives in the centre of a large town he will often escape with comparatively little suffering unless he comes accidentally into contact with a large quantity of pollen. In cases where the patient is extremely susceptible to the action of pollen he may have the symptoms pretty fully developed even in a large town, but this is not often the case.

§ 292. When the disorder is at its height and when the susceptibility is very marked the patient will have most of the severe symptoms described above; and in some instances the dyspnœa becomes so urgent if the recumbent position is assumed that for several nights in succession he will not be able to lie down. In one case I have had under my care the dyspnœa was so severe in the early years of the attacks that the patient had to sit up for twelve or fourteen nights in succession during the hay-season. At this time the patient (a lady) lived in the country: at the present time she lives in a thickly populated suburb of Manchester, and although she has an attack of hay-fever every summer the dyspnœa is never very severe.

Generally the obstruction to the breathing attains its maximum degree of severity during the night, but may be somewhat severe during the latter part of the day after the patient has been inhaling pollen for some hours. It will, however, often vary in an apparently unaccountable manner. The reason for this variation I shall allude to presently.

§ 293. The sputa will at first be thin and frothy, and may or may not be got up with difficulty. If the quantity of pollen should rise by a sort of regular progression the sputa will gradually increase, but not always in the same ratio. In the discharge from the nares the quantity seems to be governed by the quantity of pollen inhaled; it is not so, however, in the asthmatic phase of the disorder. The reason for this difference I have never been able satisfactorily to make out.

There is also another change which occurs in the discharge from the nares in a much more marked degree than it does in that from the trachea and bronchial tubes. In the declining stage of the disorder, or even when the quantity of pollen becomes suddenly lessened for more than a couple of days, there is a marked tendency for the discharge from the nostrils to become puriform; but if by chance the patient becomes again exposed to a large quantity of pollen the discharge of thin serum will commence again and will be mingled or alternated with the muco-pus. In the asthmatic form of the disorder the same thing is seen, but by no means to the same extent, and very often some portion of the sputa will come up in the shape of small pellets of semitransparent starchy-looking material.

§ 294. I have shown at § 234 that at times the granular matter of the pollen escapes from the pollen sac and floats in the air as free granular matter. I have reason to believe that when this is the case this matter will, when inhaled, penetrate much farther into the bronchial tubes than the entire pollen grain will, and that it causes less catarrh but more severe asthmatic symptoms than the pollen does. I have never, for obvious reasons, been able to demonstrate this very clearly, and can only therefore give it as an opinion which I have not as yet been able to verify; but if the opinion is correct it will help us to account for the differences we find in the severity of the asthmatic symptoms at various times, and which the quantity of pollen in the air does not always quite account for.

The duration of these symptoms will be found to differ much in different cases, and although a rapid improvement may often take place up to a certain point, some degree of obstruction in the breathing is apt to remain after most of the other symptoms have disappeared, and I believe that this is more likely to be the case when free granular matter has been inhaled than it is under other circumstances. So much, however, depends upon accidental conditions, of the precise nature of which we have not yet a full knowledge, that no rule can, at present, be laid down.

§ 295. The cough varies in character and severity in different individuals as much as any other symptom; in some cases it may be dry and spasmodic, and at the same time very troublesome; whilst in others it will be moist and will give comparatively little trouble. In some instances it is most severe in the daytime, in others in the night; and as I have before stated is attended with a varying amount of expectoration, the quantity of which seems to depend more upon the susceptibility of the mucous membrane to the influence of pollen than it does on any other circumstance; that is to say, changes of temperature, or a dry or moist condition of the atmosphere, do not seem to have much influence upon the quantity which is voided.

The condition of the urine in attacks of hay-fever has not been examined sufficiently often to permit precise statements upon it to be made. By some it is said to be quite clear and in every respect natural and healthy looking during an attack; by others it is said to be high coloured and to leave a sediment on standing.

§ 296. The general symptoms of hay-fever are differently stated by different authors. As it rarely happens that all that may occur are present in any one case this may account for the different statements made. In some instances they are almost entirely wanting, and I cannot but think the symptoms described by some patients have been due to influences which have no connection with hay-fever. When general symptoms are present they are partly due to derangement of the nervous system and partly to a disturbance in the circulation. Amongst those due to the former cause are low spirits, gloomy forebodings, a dislike to mental and physicial exertion, with a feeling of relaxation and weakness. In some cases there are pains of a neuralgic or rheumatic character in various parts of the body such as I have already alluded to as occurring in the eyeballs, orbit, and within the cranium.

In the experiments cited at §§ 138 and 139, when the arm and leg were inoculated with pollen, no pain was felt; but in some experiments subsequently tried sharp neuralgic pains were felt in the thumb and index finger of the limb operated upon and also along the course of the radial nerve.

§ 297. Dr. Phœbus says, "Dr. Cornaz mentions a lady who felt such violent pains, resembling those of rheumatism, that she was obliged to keep in bed. These were felt first in the right abdomen, then in the chest, back, in the back part of the head, especially close to the ears: these symptoms lasted the whole of the day and produced during the time a strong nervous tension in the head, back, and legs, with a difficulty of keeping the eyes open."

There is said to be a very curious state of the nervous system present in some cases where the imagination seems to be very powerful. In one case, quoted by Dr. Phœbus, the patient had an attack of sneezing with other symptoms of hay-fever "whilst looking at a beautiful picture of a hay-field." Another patient "on thinking of the disease and seeing his swollen face in the glass had all the symptoms."* I have myself never seen a patient with such

* *Der Typische Fruhsommer Katarrh oder das sogennannte Heufieber, Heu-Asthma*, p. 30.

extreme susceptibility of the nervous system as is here described, and can, therefore, only give these cases on the authority of the writers mentioned by Dr. Phœbus.

§ 298. A feverish condition, as I have previously intimated, is rarely seen in any but the asthmatic form of the disorder; except when produced artificially by inhaling pollen* or by inoculating with it, I have myself never had any feverish symptoms. When it does come on there is a frequent and full pulse, with more or less shivering; hot dry skin, with a bruised feeling in various parts of the body; sleeplessness from a crowd of ideas which will rush through the mind in spite of the patient's efforts to quiet himself and sink off to rest. These symptoms usually pass off with a profuse perspiration which may last for some hours. In the long and violent attacks of sneezing, which occur just before the hay-grass commences to be cut, the pulse will rise, the face will flush, and the respiration will quicken; but these symptoms are only temporary; in a few minutes at most they usually pass away, and do not reappear until the next paroxysm of sneezing comes on. A fit of this sort generally ends with slight shivering and with the patient being bathed all over with cold perspiration.

Although I have stated that feverish symptoms do not usually come on in the catarrhal form of the disorder, it is only right to say that I do not consider that sufficient evidence has yet been gathered on this point to enable us to say under what precise circumstances they do or do not come on. Not only is there a different amount of susceptibility in different individuals, but, if ever the matter is more closely investigated, different pollens will probably be found to have different powers in respect to the intensity of the feverish symptoms they may produce.

§ 299. Almost all authors agree in the opinion that hay-fever leaves no perceptible effects behind. It may disappear slowly in some cases, and in some it may terminate with a somewhat troublesome attack of diarrhœa, and in

---

* In these cases it was only when the pollen of one of the Amentaceæ was used that feverish symptoms came on.

others by a fit of constipation; but after the disease has once fairly passed away no sign of organic change is seen in the parts which have been affected. The eye, which may be considered one of the most highly endowed and sensitive of all organs which are attacked, recovers its healthy condition almost as quickly as any, and never, so far as I am aware, exhibits any trace of organic change in any part of its structure. Even in those cases where the asthmatic attacks have been very severe, and after they have occurred periodically for years, emphysema of the lung, which is so apt to come on in the course of long-continued attacks of ordinary asthma, is rarely, if ever, seen to follow hay-asthma.

§ 300. Hay-fever is said to be made up of two principal forms of derangement of healthy action, namely, catarrh and spasm; the former affecting all the mucous membranes with which pollen comes in contact, the latter only the muscular apparatus of the bronchial tubes. Dr. Phœbus, when referring to the asthmatic form of the disease, calls it a "laryngo-bronchio-catarrh." This designation is the best that has yet been given. Catarrh the disorder undoubtedly is in all its phases, but as regards the existence of spasm in the asthmatic form, I think I shall be able to show that this is at least very doubtful, if not impossible. To the consideration of this question I shall return presently.

In studying the nature of the disorder and in observing the changes which the affected parts undergo in its course, the question as to whether hay-fever is in any degree inflammatory naturally occurs. In considering this question we shall have to look at the mode in which pollen affects different tissues. Its leading and principal action is to produce effusion, but that this cannot always be considered inflammatory I think I shall be able to show.

§ 301. When a part is inflamed and "when liquor sanguinis is exuded it generally coagulates and constitutes a foreign body in the texture of the parts affected, which it becomes the object of nature to remove from the system, or so to modify that its presence may be rendered conducive to the wants of the economy. In order to accomplish this two kinds of changes may take place,—1st, the exudation serves as a blastema in which new vital structures originate and are developed; 2nd, it exhibits no power of becoming organized, and the exuded matters, together with the textures involved in them, die."*

In the experiments on the action of pollen on the skin, as we have seen, neither of these events came to pass. The effused fluid probably consists only of serum, and as it does not give rise to either pain, heat, or redness, and leaves no mark of its presence behind it after the exudation has been absorbed, it cannot be considered inflammatory in the proper sense of the term.

Serous exudation is said to be caused either by too great a pressure of the blood, by the want of the proper power of absorption by the lymphatics, by a watery state of the blood, or by an abnormal degree of porosity of the vessels. Since we cannot suppose that the effusion, in cases of hay-fever, is produced by any of the three first-named causes, we must believe it to be due to the abnormal porosity of the vessels.

It is a remarkable fact that when pollen is applied to the abraded skin the capillaries of the corium—the part to which the pollen is directly applied—escape its action altogether, the whole of its power being concentrated on the capillaries of the cellular tissue underneath. *It is this power of dilating, and of causing exudation from, the capillary vessels of the connective tissue that constitutes the great peculiarity in the action of pollen.*

§ 302. When pollen comes in contact with mucous membrane we have not only exudation into the submucous tissue, but also a largely increased secretion on the surface of the membrane and in its follicles; and I am inclined to think that the relative quantity of fluid poured out in these situations will vary according to the kind and condition of the pollen. In the effusion which occurs on the surface and in the effect which the effused fluid has we have phe-

* *Clinical Lectures on the Principles and Practice of Medicine*, by John Hughes Bennett, M.D., F.R.S.E., Edinburgh, 1858, p. 133.

nomena of a totally different character to those seen in the skin.

When fresh pollen is applied to the lining membrane of the nares its first effect, as I have before stated, is to produce itching; this is rapidly followed by sneezing and discharge of serum. The first contact of pollen with the Schneiderian membrane does not, so far as my experiments upon myself enable me to decide, seem to produce any inflammatory action; it is only when the discharge of serum has gone on for a time that redness and excoriation are seen. It is true that a different effect is seen when pollen is applied to the eye, but this, I think, is, as I have before intimated, partly due to mechanical irritation. If it were possible to apply pollen to the mucous membrane of the nares without producing a discharge of serum, I believe that, although we might have sneezing and also infiltration into the cellular tissue, we should have little or no inflammatory action. I have, on two or three occasions, been able to produce effusion into the submucous tissue by the application of pollen which had been reduced to a pulp by being rubbed up with water, but in these cases there was little or no sneezing at the commencement, and scarcely any discharge from the nostrils, whilst at the same time there was neither redness nor excoriation seen in any of the experiments. It is, however, only right to say that my examinations and experiments on this point have never been made in any case but my own, and cannot therefore be considered sufficient to decide the question. But whatever may be the effect which pollen has in the majority of cases when first applied, there can be no doubt about the effect which a constant discharge of fluid has upon the mucous membrane and skin over which it passes, namely, that it produces redness and excoriation.

§ 303. The exudation in the nares at first consists of a thin serum, which contains a large number of minute granules: these may generally be seen to have a vigorous molecular motion. Some part of the molecules are, no doubt, derived from the pollen grain. Interspersed with these are a number of bodies which to me look like enlarged free nuclei from pus-cells. In some of these the outline is irregular, as if there was some attempt at division, but in others the outline is circular. If dyed (on Beale's method) with an ammoniacal solution of carmine, or, better still, with a weak alcoholic solution of chloride of aniline, they are very distinctly seen on account of the avidity with which they seize upon the colouring matter; in this respect they closely resemble the nuclei of pus-cells. After the exudation has continued for a short time, cells which are not easily distinguished from the white cells of the blood are intermingled with the nuclei. Still later perfect pus-cells are present, but these are at first very few in number. In the earliest stage epithelial cells may be seen here and there, and generally these are of the ciliated kind.

After the irritation has been kept up for a length of time by the constant inhalation of pollen, very few cells of any kind will be seen in the effused fluid, the principal ingredient being the granular matter of which I have just spoken. It should be observed, however, that a single drop of the exudation will make three or four microscopic cells—each containing 700 or 800 " fields "—and that, as the character of the exuded fluid varies at different parts of the day, it would require a much greater amount of time than I could spare to enable me to say definitely what its constituents are.

§ 304. When the pollen in the air begins to diminish the number of pus-cells in a given quantity of the effusion increases, but whether it is because they are formed more rapidly, or because they are carried away less rapidly by the diminished discharge, it is impossible to say, but certain it is that, relatively to the amount of the discharge, they continue to increase until the patient becomes nearly well. It is a singular circumstance, too, that in all my examinations of the effused fluid by the microscope I have seen very few perfect pollen grains; and compared with the number inhaled, very few empty pollen sacs. Whether this must be attributed to the solvent power of the serum, or to the fact that they are to a large extent carried away by it, cannot be determined; but if I had depended upon my examinations of the exuded fluid for a knowledge of the exciting causes of hay-fever, I should have been a long time in getting any clear notion of their nature.

§ 305. The condition of the mucous membrane of the nares during attacks of hay-fever is not very easily ascertained, because that part of it with which the great bulk of the pollen comes in contact is out of sight, and probably this particular part is that which is most sensitive to its action. The part that can be seen is not at first reddened, but, as I have before observed, when the discharge has continued for a time, a diffused blush of redness may be seen, and if the quantity of pollen increases, the redness and irritation may increase until the membrane becomes very tender to the touch, from the fact of its being partially denuded of its epithelium, and also from the circumstance that the membrane itself becomes swollen and inflamed. It is said that in severe attacks of common coryza flakes of epithelium may often be found in the effused fluid. It is not the case in catarrhus æstivus, so far, at any rate, as my examinations have enabled me to decide. The quantity of the fluid effused and the length of the time that this comes away are such that it would take an enormous quantity of epithelium if only a very small amount must be present in each portion of the exudation. No doubt epithelium is formed and carried off again in some stages of the disorder, but I do not think it ever comes away in the form it is said to do in ordinary catarrh.

§ 306. When pollen ceases to be inhaled the mucous membranes soon take on the healing process; in mild cases this will be very rapid, but in cases where there has been considerable swelling and inflammation of the substance of the membrane, the change to the normal condition will be comparatively slow, and will be much the same as is seen in severe cases of ordinary catarrh. I have sometimes thought that, when the mucous membrane of the nares has been inflamed from continuous exposure to pollen for some time, a slight exposure to change of temperature from heat to cold has made the symptoms much more severe for a time. It is, however, very difficult to say when such an exposure does increase the suffering from summer catarrh, because in the latter stages of this disorder we have no means of distinguishing it from ordinary catarrh, and after the attack has passed away there is, in the condition of the mucous membrane of a hay-fever patient, nothing to show that the part has been affected, nor yet to indicate that the susceptibility still remains.

§ 307. One part of the effect produced by pollen is due to its direct action, and another to its indirect or reflex action. The discharge of serum in the nares is an example of the first kind, whilst the effusion into the subcutaneous cellular tissue is an example of the second kind of action. In the congestion of the vessels of the conjunctiva we may have both kinds of action. The reflex mode of action may be exhibited by any irritant being applied to the mucous membrane of the nostrils; every aurist knows that the introduction of the catheter to the Eustachian tube will give rise to a flow of tears and to congestion of the conjunctival vessels, and I have frequently seen the application of pollen to the nares produce slight redness of the eyeball, but this has generally been when a tolerably large quantity of pollen has been applied. Another way in which reflex action may manifest itself is when the irritation in the nostril is transferred to the bronchial tubes and produces slight asthmatic symptoms; this also I have experienced on two occasions.

§ 308. Almost every writer on hay-fever has attributed the dyspnœa which occurs in the asthmatic form of the disorder to spasm of the circular muscles of the bronchial tubes. That this is at least very doubtful I think I shall be able to show.

If we breathe through a tube which has the same diameter as the trachea we find that air enters the lungs freely, and that there is apparently a certain amount of surplus space in the tube. This is proved by the circumstance that we can breathe through tubes of a much less diameter than that of the trachea without producing any unpleasant difficulty of breathing. If, instead of using a single tube the size of the trachea, we use two tubes the diameter of the bronchial tubes which form the first division of the trachea, we find the same rule holds good. If we carry the experiment still further and use tubes of a gradually decreasing diameter, we find that to bring on the amount of dyspnœa which occurs in hay-asthma, tubes of a very small diameter would have to be used, and that consequently if such a diminution in the size of the bronchial tubes is brought about, the circulur muscles must act with a force which they cannot reasonably be supposed to possess.

The free transmission of air through the trachea and bronchial tubes is the one prime condition necessary to the proper fulfilment of their function, and even if we grant that the circular muscles have some power it is difficult to understand what purpose they could serve if they could contract the bronchial tubes down to a diameter sufficiently small to produce the dyspnœa of hay-asthma. But, whatever may be the end these circular muscular fibres are destined to serve in the economy of respiration, I am satisfied they have nothing to do with the dyspnœa of hay-asthma.

§ 309. I have shown that the peculiar and distinctive action of pollen is seen in the œdema which it produces in the cellular tissue of any part to which it is applied. This I believe is the true cause of the dyspnœa of hay-asthma, and I am also inclined to think that when all the phenomena of ordinary asthma have been thoroughly investigated a similar condition will be found to be the cause of the dyspnœa in the latter disease also. How, then, are we to account for the sudden diminution which sometimes occurs, in the severity of the dyspnœa in hay-asthma—the so-called relaxation of the spasm? I will endeavour to answer this question. It has been seen that one of the most marked symptoms of the catarrhal form of hay-fever is closure of the nasal passages by the effusion of fluid into the submucous tissue, and that at times the occlusion has been so complete that no air whatever could be drawn through the passages. So complete has the stoppage sometimes been, in the experiments described, that if respiration could only have been kept up by the air which could be made to pass through the nasal apertures, death from asphyxia must have been the result.

§ 310. In those instances in which partial occlusion occurred it was only necessary to attempt, for a time, to breathe through the nares in order to produce the true asthmatic condition, so far as the dyspnœa is concerned. How, then, is the relaxation of the so-called spasm brought about? I have shown that when a patient has been in a recumbent position for a time a change from one side to the other would close the nasal aperture on the lower side, and at the same time open the upper one; but, curiously enough, if the patient placed himself on his back when the passage of fluid from one nostril to the other was only half completed, the closure of both would be almost complete, and in this state he would find it impossible to pass sufficient air through the nostrils to keep up healthy respiration. I have again and again tried the experiment of attempting to breathe through the nostrils only when they have been in this condition, and have always found that I could produce all the distress of a true asthmatic attack by keeping up the experiment for a few minutes only.

§ 311. The same swelling of the submucous tissue is present in the larynx and trachea, and probably also in the larger bronchial tubes,* and we have only to suppose that the same changes which occur in the nares take place in the larynx or at the bifurcation of the trachea, and we have all the conditions necessary for the production of a fit of asthma, apparently by spasm, and for its relief by the so-called relaxation.

Then again exacerbations of an asthmatic attack very often occur in the night; and sometimes when the day has been comparatively free from difficulty of breathing a sudden attack may come on in the night. This also I believe is often due to a change in the position and quantity of fluid in particular parts of the cellular tissue of the air passages, nor do I think it always necessary for the bronchial tubes themselves to be affected in order to produce an asthmatic

---

* It is not probable that any great quantity of pollen penetrates to the smaller bronchial tubes, because, if this were the case, such an amount of œdema would be produced that fatal consequences must often speedily ensue.

attack. If the fluid in the cellular tissue of the buccal cavity and pharynx should gravitate towards the larynx and upper part of the trachea, this, in addition to the fluid which may already be present in these parts, would be quite sufficient to bring on severe dyspnœa. Such an alteration as that described above would be most likely to occur after the patient had placed himself in the recumbent position.

§ 312. In support of the above opinions it may be observed that position is with an asthmatic patient a very important condition. In some mild attacks of hay-asthma produced artificially I found that an alteration in the position always produced a change in the breathing which was better or worse according to circumstances. Knowing that such alterations must cause an accumulation of the effused fluid in certain spots, it is easy to see that this may give rise to dyspnœa which will vary in severity and duration according to the quantity and position of the fluid; but if spasm is the sole cause of the dyspnœa it is difficult to perceive how position can affect it in the way it does.

In putting forth these opinions I am aware that I differ from most of the writers on hay-fever, but it is only after long observation and close study of all the phenomena I have endeavoured to describe that I have been led to these conclusions.

§ 313. Hitherto the disorder has had a name applied to it which was adopted when it was supposed that the emanation from hay, in the process of being made, was the principal cause of it. We have seen that wherever flowering plants can grow in sufficient numbers to throw off a large quantity of pollen, hay-fever may be produced. Would it not therefore be better to designate it by the name of the agent which is known to produce it in every country in which it has yet been seen, namely, by the terms *pollen catarrh* and *pollen asthma?*

In suggesting this name as well as in describing the investigations I have made on this subject, I have been desirous of strictly confining my attention to the phenomena of the disorder which is brought on by pollen. There may be, and probably are, other agents which may produce symptoms not unlike those of hay-fever, but until these are found it is better to concentrate our attention upon causes within our reach rather than to allow it to be dissipated by extending our investigations over too wide an area; I have done so in this case, and have not had any cause to regret the course taken.

§ 314. The treatment of hay-fever has been spoken of by some authors as being, in their hands, very successful. I regret to say that in my hands it has been very unsuccessful; nor have I ever met with a case in which I could feel sure that the administration of remedies had really produced a cure. It is true many cases are given by authors where the use of certain remedies seemed to be followed by an improvement or by a cessation of the symptoms, but in most of these cases I am convinced that the cure was due to the patients' removal beyond the reach of the cause or to the gradual diminution in the quantity of the latter. In the early part of my yearly attacks I have frequently made the same mistake, and, with the light that the experiments described in the preceding pages have thrown upon the natural history of the disease, one cannot help feeling somewhat humbled by the recollection of the ready manner in which we are sometimes led to adopt the *post hoc ergo propter hoc* mode of reasoning.

§ 315. For some years after I first began to suffer from hay-fever I tried a great number of remedies; amongst these were baths in various forms—the vapour bath, the hot-air bath, as well as the plunge and the shower bath—but none of these seemed to be of the slightest use; and, as far as I can now remember, I was using the plunge bath regularly at the time the disorder first came on. I also used a variety of remedies in the shape of drugs. These were used in various doses: some of them, even when taken in very small doses, produced effects which made me glad to put up with the annoyance occasioned by the yearly recurrence of the disorder. *Quinine* was a medicine of this sort, as were also, to a slight extent, *Arsenic* and *Nux vomica*. But no drug that I have ever tried, either upon myself or others, has seemed to be productive of any permanent benefit; the only thing I have succeeded in doing with drugs has been to palliate, and then always by local application; such as, for instance, the application of an ointment of extract of *Belladonna* or of *Opium* to the mucous membrane of the nares. My experience of these remedies is such, however, that I do not recommend them to be used if the patient can possibly get along without them. There are, however, times, in the course of a season, when the patient will be glad to purchase temporary relief at any reasonable cost in the way of a little inconvenience caused by the use of the drugs, and it is under such circumstances that their use is justifiable.

§ 316. After my experiments commenced no treatment, except such as was merely palliative, was used. It will readily be understood that in following out the investigation this was a matter of necessity; to have attempted to try the action of remedies at the same time that I was making an effort to know the nature of the cause might have rendered the latter completely abortive: thus I found myself obliged to abandon either the one or the other for a time. I therefore elected to pursue the inquiry into the causes and nature of the disorder, and to leave the attempt to discover a remedy to the time when we should have a full knowledge of these. I am at the present time engaged in experiments on the action of various agents, and hope to be successful in my search for an effectual remedy for the disorder; but as I do not know how long these may occupy me I have preferred giving the results of my investigations as far as they have gone, rather than wait for a time which may possibly be somewhat distant.

§ 317. But although treatment by the administration of drugs has been so far of very little use, there is a possibility of alleviating the disease by a suitable change of locality, and by this means of lessening the suffering. A sojourn at the sea-side is one of the best modes of palliating and often of curing the disease for the time; but it is not every sea-side district that gives the hay-fever patient relief. Any place which, though it may be on the sea coast, partakes of the character of a bay which is deeply indented into the mainland is not favorable for the prevention of hay-fever, especially if this bay is surrounded by land which is largely used for the growth of hay-grass. But the more any sea-side place has the form and character of a small island or a narrow peninsula, and the wider is the sea which surrounds either of these, the more completely will it protect the patient from attacks of hay-fever. For this reason a cruise in a yacht, which can keep well out to sea, is one of the best remedies that can be adopted; and failing this a sojourn on a small island in the open ocean is the best that can be found on land.

But wherever a patient may be, at the sea-side, if the wind is blowing from the land, and if hay-grass is in flower at the time, he will be liable to have an attack of hay-fever. It is, therefore, a matter of importance in selecting a retreat for the hay-season to find one where the prevailing winds are from the sea. It is also better to choose a place where the patient can be continually near the water, and if possible a place where the shore is backed with high cliffs, because these act as a sort of screen when a land wind is blowing.

§ 318. I am told by Americans with whom I have conversed, that the place which enjoys the greatest reputation as a place of resort for hay-fever patients in America is Fire Island.* This island is formed by a strip of land about three quarters of a mile in breadth by about twenty miles in length: it is situated on the Atlantic side of Long Island; on one side a bay (the great South Bay), about five miles wide, separates it from Long Island, and on the other side is the broad Atlantic. Scarcely anything but a coarse short marsh grass grows upon this island, and this is very rarely seen in flower in any quantity.

We have not many places on the English coast so favorably situated as Fire Island is, but nevertheless we have

---

* On Colton's map of Long Island the place is called the "Great South Beach." On the map drawn up from the United States Survey it is termed "Fire Island Beach." Amongst Americans who visit the place it is known as "Fire Island."

some which, so far as geographical position is concerned, will be found to be quite suitable. Lundy Island (near to Ilfracombe), in the Bristol Channel, would, on trial, be found to be a place where a patient would keep clear of hay-fever. In the South of England there are Lizard Point (Cornwall), the point of land near St. Mawe's, the point of land near to Her Majesty's residence at Osborne, as well as many other places on the south coast, which I think would also afford protection from the influence of pollen. Some parts of the Isle of Man, such, for instance, as the district a little beyond Port St. Mary or Port Erin (adjoining the Calf of Man), would also be very suitable. On the Welsh Coast the district near St. David's Head is also likely to be a very suitable place for hay-fever patients to pass the season of attack at. There are also some of the small islands off the West Coast of Scotland which would give complete protection from the attacks of hay-fever.

§ 319. For those who cannot go to the seaside the next best thing is to go to the centre of a large town—the larger the better, and as far as hay-fever is concerned, the more densely populated it is the better it is for the patient. If he suffers from the asthmatic form of the complaint, though a sojourn in the centre of a large town may not be a complete protection, it will generally afford great relief, and if he can keep indoors in the middle part of the day, he will suffer less than if the time is spent principally in the open air; and even in the country if the middle of the day is passed in the house the patient will suffer a great deal less than he will in the open air. High mountain lands which are used only for grazing purposes will also be good for hay-fever patients, but these are not always as much to be depended upon as a well-chosen seaside residence is. Some parts of the Highlands of Scotland, as well as some of the mountainous districts in Wales, would be found to answer pretty well.

Mount Overlook, the highest point in the Catskill range of mountains, U.S., is a place which is very favorably spoken of by several American physicians as a place of resort for hay-fever patients in America; it is about 5000 feet above the sea level.

§ 320. I have now completed the task I set myself when I commenced my investigations on the causes and nature of hay-fever. Upon the result of the inquiry the reader can now form his own opinion. To my own mind the investigation has furnished conclusive evidence that, in this country, the exciting cause of the malady, as it occurs in summer, is the pollen of the grasses and the cereals; and also of the fact that, if a patient can, at the time these are in flower, avoid the neighbourhood where they are grown, he will to a large extent escape the attacks.

I am, as I have before intimated, quite aware that other agents may yet be found to produce symptoms not unlike those of hay-fever. Amidst the great number of bodies there are with functions similar to those of pollen, it would not be surprising if we should find some that have a similar kind of action; and it is not improbable that among these we may find the exciting causes of some diseases which are far more formidable than hay-fever. To have attempted an inquiry into the nature and mode of action of even a few of these would, in addition to the work I have done, have made the task too formidable to permit me to have a chance of completing it. I have therefore preferred to keep my attention fixed upon that part of the subject which I felt was fairly within my grasp. I cannot, however, but think that for those who have the courage to enter this path of investigation, as well as the patience and the perseverance necessary to pursue it steadily, there is a rich harvest of facts waiting to be gathered.